Non-Medical Prescribing

Non-Medical Prescribing

Multi-Disciplinary Perspectives

Eleanor Bradley and Peter Nolan

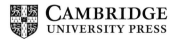

CAMBRIDGE
UNIVERSITY PRESS

CAMBRIDGE UNIVERSITY PRESS
Cambridge, New York, Melbourne, Madrid, Cape Town, Singapore, São Paulo, Delhi

Cambridge University Press
The Edinburgh Building, Cambridge CB2 8RU, UK

Published in the United States of America by Cambridge University Press, New York

www.cambridge.org
Information on this title: www.cambridge.org/9780521706872

First published 2008

Printed in the United Kingdom at the University Press, Cambridge

A catalogue record for this publication is available from the British Library

Library of Congress Cataloguing in Publication data

Bradley, Eleanor.
 Non-medical prescribing : multi-disciplinary perspectives / Eleanor Bradley and
Peter Nolan.
  p. ; cm.
 Includes bibliographical references and index.
 ISBN 978-0-521-70687-2 (pbk.)
 1. Drugs – Prescribing – Great Britain – History. 2. Nurses – Prescription privileges – Great
Britain – History. I. Nolan, Peter, lecturer in nursing studies. II. Title.
 [DNLM: 1. Prescriptions, Drug – Great Britain. 2. Nurses – trends – Great Britain.
3. Pharmacists – trends – Great Britain. 4. Professional Autonomy – Great Britain. 5. State
Medicine – trends – Great Britain. QV 748 B811n 2008]
 RM138.B73 2008
 615′.14–dc22   2008008321

ISBN 978-0-521-70687-2 paperback

For Jim and Lola

Contents

Contributors

Alan Borthwick	MSc, PhD, FChS, FHEA Lecturer at the School of Health Professions and Rehabilitation Sciences, University of Southampton Member, Medicines Committee of the Society of Chiropodists and Podiatrists
Eleanor Bradley	CPsychol, PhD, MSc, BSc (Hons) Reader in Mental Health, Faculty of Health Staffordshire University Head of R&D, South Staffordshire and Shropshire Healthcare NHS Foundation Trust
Pamela Campbell	MSc, PGCAE, RN, RM, RHV, FP Cert Primary Care Development Manager Staffordshire University Member, Advisory Panel, Queens Nursing Institute HLSP Reviewer for NMC
Amanda Evans	BPharm (Hons), Pg Dip, Postgraduate Prescribing Diploma Pharmaceutical Advisor to the provider services South Staffordshire PCT Currently undertaking PhD at Keele University
Peter Nolan	PhD, MEd, BEd (Hons), BA (Hons), RMN, RGN, DN, RNT Professor of Mental Health Nursing Staffordshire University and South Staffordshire and Shropshire Healthcare NHS Foundation Trust
Tanvir Rana	MBBS, DPM, MRC Psych Visiting Senior Lecturer in Mental Health Faculty of Health, Staffordshire University Locum Consultant Psychiatrist, South Staffordshire and Shropshire Healthcare NHS Foundation Trust

Foreword

I would like to thank Prof Peter Nolan and Dr Eleanor Bradley at Staffordshire University for the chance to contribute this foreword. Staffordshire University was one of the very first universities to offer the former 'Extended Formulary Nurse Prescribing' postgraduate course, and the first Extended Formulary Nurse Prescribers [now Nurse Independent Prescribers] qualified from there. I oversee the Non-Medical Prescribing work programme at the Department of Health, so I was both interested and pleased to see Staffordshire's work.

The publication of this book is timely. We now have nearly 10 000 Nurse Independent Prescribers, and approaching 150 Pharmacist Independent Prescribers. There are 850 Pharmacist Supplementary prescribers; and the numbers of Allied Health Professional [AHP] Supplementary Prescribers – mainly physiotherapists and chiropodists/podiatrists – continue to grow steadily.

Extending prescribing responsibilities to nurses, pharmacists and other health professionals has not only improved patients' access to medicines; it also recognises the skills of senior and highly experienced professionals. Rigorous training and assessment processes help ensure that patient safety remains paramount and that prescribers are able to deliver effective patient care in a variety of settings.

There are now nurse and pharmacist prescribers in almost all areas of the NHS – from primary care, community setting, secondary and specialist care to palliative care. As the NHS moves away from hospital-based care and closer to the patient, non-medical prescribing provides an important mechanism to help deliver that care. Nurse prescribing also underpins two of the key elements of *Modernising Nursing Careers* by helping to *develop a competent and flexible workforce* and *modernise the image of nursing and nursing careers*.

Non-medical prescribing has also encouraged multi-disciplinary team working and better communication between professions. I am very grateful to those who have given their time and skills to train Non-Medical Prescribers. In fact, the training programme would not have been possible without support from doctors. Every non-medical prescriber has benefitted from having a designated medical practitioner during their training to provide on-the-job training, and professional advice.

This book indicates that extending prescribing responsibilities has helped to enhance the existing skills that experienced nurses, pharmacists and AHPs already possess. Health professionals feel they have gained both personally and professionally from becoming prescribers.

I was particularly pleased to see that Nurse Independent Prescribers felt their communications with other prescribers had improved and that their confidence has increased around medicines. Pharmacists, although relatively new to prescribing responsibilities, have had a positive impact on patients – especially when helping patients to manage long-term conditions with complex medication regimes. This book has indicated that being able to work with patients and intervene as appropriate with their treatment, if necessary, has helped to reinvigorate the pharmacist's role. AHP Supplementary Prescribers, although still quite small in number, are making a real contribution to improving patient care – building on their existing knowledge and skills to provide treatment for whole episodes of care.

An evaluation of Nurse Prescribing in 2005 indicated that nurse prescribers were prescribing frequently and [clinically] appropriately.[1] Feedback from patients about nurse prescribing was also positive. DH is now commissioning further work to evaluate Nurse and Pharmacist Independent Prescribing – beginning in 2008. I believe it is important to assess policy after implementation because evaluation provides us with a means to hone the policy further and help provide the best solution for patients.

Non-Medical Prescribing is a mechanism to draw on what can help improve NHS services for patients. I accept that, in some areas, there is still work needed and that there are still some issues to resolve, especially at a local, grassroots level. But I am heartened to see that Non-Medical Prescribing has had a positive impact, with both patients and professionals satisfied.

Professor Christine Beasley
Chief Nursing Officer
Department of Health, England

[1] 'Evaluation of extended formulary independent nurse prescribing', Prof S. Latter, University of Southampton, 27th June 2005.

Preface

Terminology

Throughout this book, the terminology for prescribing by nurses and other professions allied to health varies from non-medical prescribing, to nurse prescribing, to non-doctor prescribing. In all these cases, the authors are referring to instances in which professionals other than doctors are able to prescribe medicines. The phrase 'nurse prescribing' is problematic as it excludes other professions, such as those allied to medicine, that are now able to prescribe medicines. However, the research findings described in Chapters 3, 4 and 5 were drawn from a study that was completed only with nurses (because only nurses were permitted to prescribe at the beginning of the project), so this research commonly refers to nurse prescribing. The term 'non-medical prescribing' has been widely adopted and is used throughout the Department of Health (DoH) policy documents. However, this term has come in for some criticism from professionals, who consider all prescribing to be an inherently 'medical' activity and that therefore all prescribers are 'medical' prescribers, even if they are not medics. To counter this issue, a preferred terminology is 'non-doctor prescribing', and this term has been used as appropriate throughout this text.

Guide to prescribing in the UK

To preface the chapters in this book, a brief guide to the types of prescribing available to non-doctor prescribers in the UK is provided. However, more detailed accounts of the development of non-doctor prescribing in the UK and fuller definitions and discussions of the different types of prescribing than can be found here are outlined in other texts (e.g. Courtney and Griffiths, 2004).

Community nurses have been able to prescribe from a limited formulary of medication (Nurse Prescribers' Formulary [NPF]) for over 20 years in the UK. In April 2003, prescribing rights were extended to specially trained nurses working in other specialities, permitting nurses to prescribe as independent prescribers from a limited list in the British National Formulary (BNF) for a specified list of conditions (DoH, 2002). Supplementary prescribing was also introduced for nurses and pharmacists, permitting them to prescribe any drug from the BNF provided that they were working from a clinical management plan (CMP) for that specific service user that has been fully agreed with a medical practitioner (DoH, 2002). In May 2005, supplementary prescribing was extended to physiotherapists, chiropodists/podiatrists, radiographers and optometrists. In May 2006, the independent prescribing initiative was extended, and qualified nurse independent prescribers were able to prescribe any licensed medicine, including some controlled drugs, for any medical condition within their competence. On the same date, the availability of prescribing for pharmacists was extended, permitting pharmacist independent prescribers to prescribe any licensed medicine, with the exception of controlled drugs, for any medical condition within their competence (DoH, 2006).

REFERENCES

Courtenay, M. & Griffiths, M. (2004) *Independent and Supplementary Prescribing: An Essential Guide.* Cambridge, UK: Cambridge University Press.

Department of Health (2002) Nurses will prescribe for chronic illness says Professor David Haslam. Press Release, 2002/0488, 21 November. London: Department of Health.

Department of Health (2006) http://www.dh.gov.uk/en/Policyandguidance/ Medicinespharmacyandindustry/Prescriptions/ TheNon-MedicalPrescribingProgramme/Nurseprescribing/index.htm.

Acknowledgements

A considerable debt of gratitude is due to the many institutions and people who contributed to bringing this project to fruition. First and foremost, we would like to acknowledge the funding provided by Pfizer Ltd. and the interest it has shown in the project, particularly by John Bayliss. We also express our thanks to the former Workforce Development Directorate in Staffordshire and Shropshire, to Carole Blackshaw, in particular, and to the former South Staffordshire Mental Health Trust. Staffordshire University has also taken a keen interest in the project and has been generous with its support throughout. We are mindful of the various Ethical Committees and Nurse Prescribing Leads with whom we have worked; they provided invaluable advice, suggestions and information. The Non-Medical Prescribing Module Leaders at the Universities of Coventry, Worcester, Central England, Wolverhampton and Staffordshire were superb in assisting us with data collection. We express our gratitude to Dr Sayeed Haque, Health Statistician at Birmingham University, for his vital contribution to the study.

Special mention must be made of Neil Carr, OBE, Chief Executive of South Staffordshire and Shropshire NHS Foundation Trust, who has tirelessly championed non-medical prescribing in the West Midlands. He has been keen to use the findings from the study on which this book is based to ensure that the introduction of non-medical prescribing was planned and informed, as well as sensitively and effectively deployed.

Finally, without the contributions of the nurse prescribers, who readily and generously gave of their time, the study and this book would not have been possible. At a time when healthcare personnel are so often the subject of criticism, the testimonies and accounts of service users of the amazing care they have received were both enlightening and humbling.

Eleanor Bradley and Peter Nolan

Introduction

Peter Nolan and Eleanor Bradley

Among the many innovations in healthcare that came to the fore in the UK during the first decade of the twenty-first century was legislation allowing professionals other than doctors to prescribe for patients under certain conditions. Non-medical prescribing, as it is generally referred to, has been the focus of research, commentary and debate for some time. Although the number of prescribers has been growing steadily, those who opt to take on this role are still a minority within their respective professions. Some commentators have played down its significance; but others have seen it as symptomatic of a radically changing National Health Service (NHS) and a predictor of many more radical changes to come. There is little doubt that non-medical prescribing has the potential to change the concept and delivery of healthcare provision in the UK.

The idea of granting professions other than the medical profession prescriptive authority was first mooted in the UK in 1986. Although non-medical prescribing was initially restricted to community nurses, it has gathered rapid momentum during the first decade of the twenty-first century and has now extended to many more disciplines (Humphries & Green, 2002). Although time and resources were required to prepare personnel for prescribing, it was generally believed that the advantages of having non-medical prescribers would more than compensate for the effort of training them. Non-medical prescribers would, it was argued, provide more choice for patients and encourage well-informed debate about the benefits and drawbacks of pharmacological interventions (Luker *et al.*, 1998). It was hoped that non-medical prescribers would have more time to guide, support, review and monitor patients, with the potential for the public to be better educated about its medicines, more capable of making informed decisions about medicine-taking and more responsive to the need to adhere to treatment regimens. Furthermore, it was intended that non-medical prescribing would bring together doctors, pharmacists, nurses and patients so that the prescribing process would be better informed and more appropriate than it had been in the past.

Non-medical prescribing seemed, on many counts, to be a very worthwhile development during a period when healthcare was high on the political agenda. Policy documents produced by the Department of Health (DoH, 2001a, 2001b, 2005) stated that people had a right to high-quality care, provided at a time that suited them and in a way that best met their needs. People's expectations were heightened by periodic reports of medical progress which promised they could be spared from suffering, live longer, happier lives and be more fulfilled in everything they did. The centrality of service users to healthcare delivery was repeatedly emphasised, and 'expert patients', 'patient advocates' and 'patient champions' became the reference points for establishing and evaluating services. Public expectations were deliberately heightened as a means of ensuring that services would improve. Implicit in government's thinking was the assumption that people had the right to the best treatments and the best medicines, regardless of cost, and that individuals could expect to be able to avail themselves of whatever was considered to be the best. Ager (2007) claimed that while there was good practice in relation to prescribing in the UK, it generally lagged behind the rest of Europe in terms of getting newer and better drugs to patients faster, especially in the areas of cancer, cardiac disease and HIV.

As the debate about how medicines should be regulated and utilised continued, it became apparent that heightening people's expectations could lead to two unintended consequences: patients might make excessive demands on staff for specific medicines and could demand medicines that were not necessarily in their best interests. Rose (2007) noted that 14.7 million prescriptions were written for antidepressants in 2005 and that this number increased to 31 million in 2006, costing the NHS £291.5 million. Many doctors agreed that they were prescribing antidepressants too readily but claimed that their practice was being dictated by patients who wanted medication, and who could not be referred to alternative behavioural or counselling treatments because of their lack of availability. As far back as 1985, Vaillant and Perry (1985) had questioned the assumption that medicines provide 'better living through biochemistry' and had suggested that pharmacotherapy was best used sparingly.

These problems are not unique to the United Kingdom. The World Health Organisation (WHO, 2003) has stressed that merely making medicines available does not equate with instant health gain, especially if patients do not take their medications in accordance with how they should be taken. The same document noted that, in developed countries, only 50% of patients suffering from chronic disease adhere to treatment recommendations and that older people consume approximately 60% of medicines (three times that of the general population), even though they make up less than 20% of the population. The report recommended paying greater attention to:

patient education, health education, assisting people to address their own needs, the provision of more supportive consultations, the availability of better screening for co-morbidity and paying greater attention to those with mental health problems. (WHO, page 72)

The importance of working with patients was emphasised by Horne and Weinman (1999), who concluded that failure to take into account the beliefs and values of patients would make it likely that any medicines prescribed would not be taken appropriately.

In 2004, WHO was concerned that people were taking drugs that did not directly address their health needs. It was noted that while the Internet played an important part in the distribution of medical products, it also led to people being put at risk because they were taking drugs without having information about their possible side effects or associated dangers. This applied both to therapeutic medicines and, perhaps even more so, to lifestyle medicines:

The greatest areas of risk concern lifestyle drugs such as anabolic steroids, drugs for weight loss and hair loss. To maintain public confidence in the health care system, it is necessary to prevent unreliable products from entering the internet which is by definition a highly volatile mechanism for mass-border trade and difficult to police. (WHO, 2004, p. 152)

A few years earlier, WHO (2001) had also raised concerns about complementary and traditional medicines. It recommended that each country should be alert to the increase in the number of outlets for such medicines and the need to protect people as much as possible, although acknowledging that these medicines had the potential to improve quality of life, even if they could not cure diseases such as cancer or AIDS.

Modernisation

The rise of non-medical prescribing coincided with the establishment of the NHS Modernisation Agency in 2001, which had the task of coordinating the vast array of changes then taking place. This was a frantic period in the history of the NHS, when multiple policies were being implemented simultaneously. Central to the philosophy of modernisation were transparency, new ways of working and payment by results. It was felt that what the NHS required was not more staff but to make better use of those already in post, and this meant breaking down barriers between professions to allow duties traditionally undertaken by one group to be carried out by others. Role redesign and new ways of working became a priority because flexibility would enable staff to collaborate with other disciplines in order to respond to advances in medical knowledge and technologies and to the demands of the public for better integrated and more convenient healthcare.

Other developments directly and indirectly related to the emergence of non-medical prescribing included the reduction in doctors' working hours (due to be fully implemented by 2009), an increased involvement of patients and carers in their own care and the democratisation of information. Just as important were social reforms and changes in British consciousness, which were tending towards a more egalitarian society in which inherited privilege and traditional roles were being questioned. The context within which non-medical prescribing evolved was therefore one of challenge to traditional medical hegemony and increasing public assertiveness about its healthcare requirements.

Nurses are, and have been, the largest group of non-medical prescribers in the NHS. The nature and extent of the work they have been undertaking has been changing rapidly and radically. The authority to prescribe is not an end in itself but a component of nurses' newly emerging roles. For instance, neonatal nurses are increasingly taking on duties formerly performed by junior doctors, and many are highly skilled in the technologies associated with special care baby units. As prescribers, they review treatment regimens for at-risk babies, monitor them and, when necessary, change treatment and medicines. Similarly, nurses working in plastic and cardiac surgery are now removing 'lumps and bumps' and 'vein stripping'; there are few whose role would be no more than that of the traditional theatre nurse. Clinical nurse specialists have retained much of their nursing role but also provide extensive advice and support to patients, and many have become independent prescribers in order to provide appropriate and timely treatment for patients. Respiratory nurses run asthma clinics and keep patients out of hospital by developing clinical management plans (CMPs), monitoring treatments and prescribing independently. They also lead ward rounds and provide in- and out-patient management and advice. At the beginning of their treatment journey, cardiology patients meet nurses who clerk them in and can manage the supply, administration and prescribing of medication via Patient Group Directions (PGDs). Patients will not see a doctor until they are in the catheter lab. This has resulted in more patients being able to access cardiology services and being seen faster.

Problems around role creation

It seems probable that introducing change based on twenty-first century thinking into a system that had existed for well over half a century and in which professionals' roles have never been critically examined would result either in resistance or failure. There has certainly been some resistance; it remains to be seen whether non-medical prescribing can achieve what it was intended to do.

The role of non-medical prescriber is not conferred as a result of experience but by completing a course and undertaking a period of supervised practice. Educational courses have been the traditional way of attempting to redesign roles, and the usual mode of educational provision is through classroom-based learning. Little guidance was given as to the selection of candidates for non-medical prescribing training or about the prescribing roles they are expected to take on once qualified. From the start of the initiative, those who elected to become prescribers did so voluntarily. Corrigan *et al.* (2001) noted, not surprisingly, that merely sending people on a course did not guarantee that they could put an entirely new role into operation. These researchers found that some students elected to go on courses primarily because they were not coping with their jobs or were close to burnout. Certain services, they argued, were unlikely to welcome a clinician in a new role unless all those who worked in the team had been involved in designing the role and were fully supportive of the person taking it on. Lightfoot and Orford (1986) argued that training for new roles must increase motivation, address role ambiguity and enhance role legitimacy. It has been found that where staff undertaking new roles are unsupported, as many as 50% leave within 18 months (Graham *et al.*, 2006). To avoid this happening, people must feel they have adequate knowledge and skills to do the job; they must be able to work with others and feel supported in order to ensure their self-esteem. Corrigan and McCracken (1995) suggest that implementation of training is more likely to be effective if this task is seen as belonging not to the individual but to the whole team.

The aims of this book, and the contribution it seeks to make, are to explore how non-medical prescribing is affecting practice and the experiences and observations of those directly involved in its implementation. Furthermore, it seeks to provide an account of how one development in healthcare, albeit an important one, was approached in one part of the country, and, hopefully, it will prove valuable not only to those currently working in healthcare but also to future commentators on health services. What differentiates this book from other texts is that it brings together observation and commentaries of more than one prescribing group. What transpires within healthcare is open to multiple interpretations, and the introduction of non-medical prescribing is no exception.

Chapter 1 takes a broad-brush approach to the evolution of the prescribing of medicines and in doing so shows that many of the concerns and themes present in today's NHS proved problematic for our predecessors also. Similar concerns have arisen in the past with respect to issues such as: What constitutes a medicine? What constitutes evidence of efficacy? and Under what conditions are people permitted to have access to medicine? Different societies at different times have responded in varying ways depending on the social, political and economic climates of the time, coupled with the power possessed by the healthcare elites. This chapter explores how our society is responding to these and other concerns relating to the prescribing of medicines at this time. Chapter 2 provides an in-depth account of how nurses came to be involved in prescribing and the many and varied stages that were required to make it a reality. Chapter 3 examines the characteristics of nurses who opted to train as prescribers between 2003 and 2006, particularly their backgrounds, reasons for opting to train as prescribers and perceptions of the potential impact of future prescribing roles. Chapter 4 utilises data gathered from recently qualified nurse prescribers to highlight the impact that prescribing has had in practice, the barriers to prescribing and some of the key benefits to prescribing. Chapter 5 describes how the rollout of non-medical prescribing has been perceived by healthcare teams, doctors and service users, outlining experiences of working alongside, and being treated by, non-medical prescribers, as well as more general attitudes towards the non-medical prescribing initiative itself and the potential impact it could have on professional roles. Chapter 6 presents an analysis of how prescribing pharmacists are involved in prescribing, how they view prescribing generally, how it benefits patients and their carers, how they relate to other members of their team and how it could alter the role of pharmacists in the future. An extensive overview is presented in Chapter 7 of five groups of allied health professionals: podiatrists, physiotherapists, radiographers, optometrists and ambulance paramedics. Special attention is given to how these groups are utilising prescribing as part of their practice and how the services they provide for their patients are changing. Finally, Chapter 8 draws conclusions from the previous chapters. It highlights the lessons learned so far about the implementation of non-medical prescribing and makes some cautious recommendations about future directions and requirements.

It addition to informing readers, it is hoped that the following chapters will challenge, provoke and incline them to consider deeply what is currently taking place within health services and the many and varied ways in which traditional roles are being overhauled and redesigned.

REFERENCES

Ager, B. (2007) The research-based pharmaceutical industry – a key actor for a healthy Europe. *The Official Hope Reference Book.* London: Camden Publishing Limited.

Cartwright, A. K., Hyams, G. & Spratley, T. (1996) Is the interviewer's therapeutic commitment an important factor in determining whether alcoholic clients engage with treatment? *Addiction Research*, **4**, 215–30.

Corrigan, P. W. & McCracken, S. G. (1995) Refocusing the training of psychiatric rehabilitation staff. *Psychiatric Services*, **46**, 1172–7.

Corrigan, P. W., Steiner, L., McCracken, S. G. *et al.* (2001) Strategies for disseminating evidence-based practices to staff who treat people with serious mental illness. *Psychiatric Services*, **52**, 1598–606.

Department of Health (2001a) *Investment and Reform for NHS Staff – Taking Forward the NHS Plan.* London: Department of Health.

Department of Health (2001b) Patients get quicker access to medicines. Press release: reference 2001/0223. London: Department of Health.

Department of Health (2005) *Creating a Patient-Led NHS.* London: Department of Health.

Department of Health (2006) *Medicines Matters: A Guide to Mechanisms for the Prescribing, Supply and Administration of Medicines.* London: Department of Health.

Graham, I., Fielding, C., Rooke, D. & Keen, S. (2006) Practice Development 'without walls' and the quandary of corporate practice. *Journal of Clinical Nursing,* **15**(8), 980–8.

Humphries, J. L. & Green, E. (2000) Nurse prescribers: infrastructures required to support their role. *Nursing Standard,* **14**(48), 35–9.

Horne, R. & Weinman, J. (1999) Patients' beliefs about prescribed medicines and their role in adherence to treatment in chronic physical illness. *Journal of Psychosomatic Research,* **47**(6), 555–67.

Lightfoot, P. J. & Orford, J. (1986) Helping agents' attitudes towards alcohol-related problems: situation vacant: a test and elaboration of a model. *British Journal of Addiction,* **81**, 749–56.

Luker, K. A., Austin, L., Hogg, C., Fergison, B. & Smith, K. (1998) Nurse-patient relationships: the context of nurse prescribing. *Journal of Advanced Nursing,* **28**, 235–42.

Rose, D. (2007) Britian becomes a Prozac nation. *The London Times,* 14 May, p. 1.

Vaillant, G. E. & Perry, J. C. (1985) Personality disorders. In: Kaplan, H. & Sadock, B. (eds), *Comprehensive Textbook of Psychiatry.* Baltimore: Williams & Wilkins, p. 958–68.

World Health Organisation (2001) Wilson, W. (ed), *General Guidelines for Methodologies on Research and Evaluation of Traditional Medicine.* Geneva: WHO.

World Health Organisation (2003) Sabate, S. (ed), *Adherence to Long-term Therapies.* Geneva: WHO.

World Health Organisation (2004) WHO Drug Information, vol 18, no 1. Geneva: WHO.

1

Medicines and prescribing – past and present

Peter Nolan and Eleanor Bradley

Wherever human communities have existed, strong evidence suggests that they used an assortment of medicines for alleviating suffering and promoting health (Wear, 1992). Healthcare in the past was closely aligned to the environment in which people lived, and being close to nature contributed to the health and well-being of individuals as well as the prosperity and survival of the tribe. Medicines were dispensed and administered by healers and shamans, who were revered for their skills in combating the malevolent forces thought to cause disease (Sonnedecker, 1976). Their medicines, often referred to as 'nostrums' (Latin *nostrum remedium*, meaning 'our remedy'), were developed from a profound knowledge of plants, herbs and minerals. Healers strove to keep the constituents of their medicines secret from other tribes and healers. To enhance their thera-peutic potency, medicines had to be administered under special conditions that might relate to the time of day or phase of the moon and, in addition, were usually accompanied by elaborate rituals, incantations and prayers. In various forms, natural remedies have doubtless brought comfort to countless millions over the centuries, and people have continued to believe in them despite the fact that they have sometimes proved disappointing or even lethal in their effects (Parish 1980). Today it is known that a number of factors beyond the con-stituents of the medicinal compound itself contribute to the benefit derived from them; these factors include being clear about what the problem is, trusting the person who prescribes the treatment and abiding by whatever regimens or lifestyle changes are recommended in order to restore and promote health.

The history of modern pharmacy has been traced back to the peoples of Mesopotamia, who lived in the valleys of the Nile, Tigris and the Euphrates Rivers several thousand years before Christ. These fertile valleys allowed the cul-tivation of an array of herbs and plants; the medicaments and nostrums derived from these are still in use today. Arabic healers made a major contribution to the development of pharmacy by systematically recording how medicines were made and administered. This documentation, preserved and developed over decades, was brought together as the *Pharmakon* (Wertenbaker, 1980), a handbook in which medicines for every known malady were described in extraordinary detail, along with their methods of administration and the durations of treatment (Campbell, 1926). Excavators of the tomb of Sennacherib, king of Assyria (883–858 B.C.), found 250 vegetable-based and 120 mineral-based drugs as well as other therapeutic preparations containing alcohol, fats, honey, milk and wax (Rawcliffe, 1999). It would appear that medicines played such an important part in the ancient world that they were buried with the great and powerful to give them comfort in the afterlife. Centuries-old wisdom relating to health maintenance is still reflected in the culture and practices of illiterate nomadic peoples such as the Bedouins in the Sinai Peninsula and the Berbers in North Africa. Without specialist organisations or personnel to deliver health services, these tribes rely on transmitting their understanding of how to live healthily from one generation to the next.

In ancient Egypt, healing education took place in the temples in Memphis, Thebes and Heliopolis, which were referred to as 'houses of life'. Here, medicine and pharmacy were taught, and those with an honest character and the appropriate scientific background were chosen to become teachers and professors in the schools (Nunn, 1996). The principal medical specialities related to abdominal and eye diseases and dentistry. Knowledge of how to treat illnesses was highly regarded, and those who practiced medicine were often seen as equal to a god (Gardiner, 1938). Eminent physicians such as Imhotep, who lived around 2630 B.C., seem not only as doctors but also as priests, magicians, scribes and philosophers (Strouhal, 1992). The physician who examined the sick had to be knowledgeable, but the pharmacists who provided the remedies were regarded even more highly for their understanding of nature and especially human nature. The books in which medical and pharmacological learning were recorded were guarded by a specially appointed priest, the 'keeper of the sacred books'.

The regulation of medicines

During the early eighth century, the Arabs conquered Spain; they remained there until the fifteenth century. This period, when Christians, Muslims and Jews lived harmoniously together, was one of great advances in healthcare. In Cordova and Toledo, Arabic healthcare texts were translated and made available to Western scholars and health practitioners, who were predominantly highly educated monks involved in the provision of healthcare to the poor and to pilgrims resting at the monasteries (Hudson, 1983). The fusion of Arabic and European thinking generated a systematic approach to illness and its treatment and a compassionate approach to care which persisted long beyond the Middle Ages (Rawcliffe, 1999).

At the beginning of the sixteenth century, healthcare and the administration of medicines began to move away from their monastic foundations. In 1511,

Thomas Linacre obtained the exclusive right to train a small group of people as secular doctors (Black, 2006). The College of Physicians was established in 1518; by the eighteenth century, there had emerged three groups of healthcare practitioners, different from each other in terms of their training, social status and income. The first of these were *physicians* or *gentlemen*, who had been educated at Oxford or Cambridge, generally in the classics or humanities, and who then went to London to gain 6 months of experience in hospital practice. On completion of their 'training', they were issued a licence that restricted them to working within 7 miles of London. These gentlemen advised rather than treated patients and saw only those who had the means to pay for their services. Doctors who elected to work unpaid in the voluntary hospitals nonetheless charged large fees, which were paid to the students who accompanied them on their rounds. Some wards had to be enlarged to accommodate the number of students attracted by famous doctors. Doctors were judged on their ability to generate income for the hospital by means of attracting either patients or students; little attention was paid to how effective they were as doctors! The second group consisted of the surgeons who treated problems such as abscesses and fractures and undertook work that required speed and dexterity. The third group comprised the apothecaries, who were lower-middle-class tradesmen and whose duties were restricted to compounding and dispensing drugs. They were the only source of medical assistance for the majority of people and were not allowed to charge for any advice given but only for the medicines they prescribed. Such was the demand for their services in comparison to those of physicians that they established their own organisation, the Society of Apothecaries, in 1774. All three groups, despite the competition between them and their different social standing, were united in their opposition to unlicensed practitioners.

At the beginning of the nineteenth century, the making and dispensing of drugs had become the province of two groups – the chemists who dealt in chemicals and the druggists who dealt in drugs of animal and vegetable origin. Both were regarded as tradesmen, not as gentlemen. In 1815, they were formally recognised in terms of their right to buy, compound, dispense and sell drugs and medicines to the public. They became members of the Society of Apothecaries alongside the apothecaries who had been giving medical advice; apothecaries who merely dispensed were excluded from membership (Porter, 1997). Advising apothecaries were to become part of the emerging medical profession, while the dispensing apothecaries later became pharmacists. Until 1841, dispensing apothecaries were trained via an apprenticeship system, usually in the form of fathers passing their trade on to their sons. Their businesses were easily identified in towns and cities by the distinctive lighting above the entrances of their premises. In addition to selling their own remedies, they also sold sauces, pickles, spices, tea, coffee, varnishes, ink, oil and tobacco (Black, 2006). In 1841, the Pharmaceutical Society of Great Britain was established with headquarters in Bloomsbury Square. Here, a school of pharmacy was established, and lectures were delivered on medical botany, chemistry, *materia medica* and pharmacy.

On 19 July 1832, the Provincial Medical and Surgical Association (PMSA), later to become the British Medical Association (BMA), was founded by Sir Charles Hastings (1794–1866) at a meeting in the boardroom of Worcester Infirmary. Its objectives were to promote the medical and allied sciences and to support the honour and interests of the medical profession. Almost immediately after its foundation, the association became involved in the struggle for medical reform which resulted, in 1858, in the passing of the Medical Act. This established the General Medical Council and the Medical Register, therefore distinguishing, for the first time, between qualified and unqualified practitioners, seeking to differentiate 'real doctors' and 'real medications' from 'quacks' and 'hoax medicines' (Porter, 2004).

The Medical Act differentiated among prescribing, dispensing and administering medicines. This division of labour, which later defined the remit of doctors, pharmacists and nurses, existed to the end of the twentieth century. In 1868, the Pharmacy Act legislated that all who registered as chemists or druggists should be appropriately trained and regulated. In 1925, the School of Pharmacy was absorbed into the University of London, and degree courses replaced the traditional apprenticeship training (Black, 2006).

An understanding of herbs and their actions was still the basis of much treatment, especially in circumstances where access to doctors and medicines was limited. During the Crimean War, Mary Seacole (1805–1881) – who had learned about herbal treatments by assisting her Jamaican mother, whom she described as an admirable doctress, in the making of tinctures, nostrums, poultices and dietary supplements – kept a boarding house for invalid soldiers. Prompted by the outbreak of cholera among the soldiers, she travelled to the Crimea with the aim of providing support for wounded and infected soldiers. She had acquired her skills and knowledge as a result of travelling widely in the Caribbean and South America, studying the medicinal properties of plants and minerals, which she wrote about in her book, first published in 1857 (Seacole, 1990). Her knowledge of herbal treatments enabled her to set about treating not only infected wounds but also other conditions such as gastritis, fevers, foot rot, lice infestation and malnutrition. She combined physical and spiritual care, making a contribution to the development of both medicine and nursing at least as great as that of Florence Nightingale. Such was the demand by the public at this time for medicines that would treat illness and improve health that John Boot, founder of the Boots chain of chemist shops, opened the first establishment that sold herbal remedies in Nottingham in 1849.

By the end of the nineteenth century, despite the plethora of drugs being prescribed and dispensed, only a very few were specific in their actions. These were digitalis for heart conditions, quinine for malaria, pecacuanha for dysentery and mercury for the treatment of syphilis. Scurvy could be treated with fruit and vegetables, toothache remedied by extraction and gangrene by amputation. Pain could be managed with laudanum, opium, alcohol and cocaine. Medicines remained largely impotent against most human maladies, and doctors doubtless killed more people than they saved (Olie & Loo, 1999). The potential market for effective drugs was clearly huge when people were prepared to continue taking even medicines which had no obvious benefits. At the start of the twentieth century, the lure of handsome profits brought into being the first great pharmaceutical companies, such as Roche, the forerunner of Ciba-Geigy, in Switzerland; Pfizer, Eli Lilly, Merck and Abbott Laboratories in the United States; and Glaxo, Beecham and the Wellcome Foundation in the UK. These companies began to produce medicines in laboratory conditions, using synthetic materials as opposed to natural ingredients, very different from how the apothecaries had traditionally produced their concoctions. Being unable to sell all their products directly to the public, the companies relied on high street and hospital pharmacists to store and dispense their products. Some of these were an improvement on what had gone before, although unpleasant side effects were common. The companies tended to play these down, with a spokesperson for Eli Lilly commenting that, 'a drug without side effects is no drug at all' (McNight, 1995).

The rise of the NHS

Black (2006) noted that the history of health and social services demonstrates considerable fluidity; they grow, divide and merge depending on demographic influences and social trends. Healthcare has been significantly influenced by pharmacology and the growth in number and expectations of the population, by the healthcare needs of migrants and by the political orientation of governments. Britain has made significant contributions to the development of healthcare worldwide, but it has also eagerly adopted ideas from abroad. Anatomical dissection as a tool for training doctors originated in France, medical societies and postgraduate medical education were copied from Italy and Vienna and nursing sisterhoods originated in Germany. Smallpox inoculation was first implemented on a wide scale in Turkey and later taken up in Britain. Healthcare institutions in the UK have always been adept at spotting progressive practices all over the world and adopting them when appropriate.

The National Health Service (NHS), established in 1948, now employs 1.3 million people and is the third-largest employer in the world. Its original aim was to centralise and coordinate the myriad health services and facilities that existed at the beginning of the twentieth century in the UK and to make treatments freely available to all in need, thus relieving people of the fear of illness and incapacity. Five years of war had resulted in an exhausted, impoverished, unhealthy and undernourished population, where basic foods such as meat, cheese, sugar and tea were rationed. Many people ate mostly bread, with large queues formed early each morning outside bakers' shops. Living conditions for large sections of the population were unpropitious. Over 12 million dwellings had no bath, hot water or inside toilet. The icy-cold winter of 1946–1947, coupled with a shortage of coal, resulted in the early demise of some while reducing others to despair (Kynaston, 2007). Many were able for the first time in their lives to see a doctor and be treated. Although the NHS was doubtless underpinned by a genuine humanitarian ethos, it was also intended to fulfil an economic imperative by creating a healthy workforce to re-establish post-war Britain as the rich and powerful nation that it had traditionally been. Health was the medium through which, it was believed, the British nation could reclaim its past glories. It was recognised that health was influenced not just by health services but also by education, housing, income, leisure and social networks; indeed, the first Minister of Health following the Second World War was also the Minister for Housing.

Aneurin Bevan, who was Minister of Health between 1945 and 1951 and also the chief architect of the NHS, argued that healthcare was fundamental to meet human needs; without it, there was uncertainty and chaos (Webster, 2002). It was more than a means of promoting and sustaining an individual's health; it was the expression of a nation's pride, a means of transforming the national economy and a badge of civilisation. Herbert Morrison (1888–1965), one of the founder members of the London Labour Party and Mayor of Hackney from 1920 to 1921, helped draft the 1945 election party manifesto that included the blueprints for nationalisation and welfare programmes. After the Labour victory, Morrison declared that wealth would no longer be the only passport to the best treatment. Rich and poor would be treated alike. Both Bevan and Morrison were confident that their socialist values could be translated into practice (Webster, 1988). Inglis (1981), however, notes that policies conceived in the rarefied atmosphere of committee rooms have to be implemented in the messy world of scarce resources and by people who may not be as well disposed towards them as those who proposed them.

Whereas the NHS was well intentioned and highly regarded by the population at large, the creation of such a vast organisation proved more challenging and expensive than the majority of politicians and planners had foreseen. The optimism which had led to the attempt to bring together diverse organisations such as Poor Law institutions, religious organisations, infirmaries, dispensaries and local authority services was soon shown to be misguided. Critics argued that it had been naïve to expect services with such varying histories, cultures, aims and management styles to abandon their respective philosophies and merge voicelessly into the NHS (Klein *et al.*, 1996).

Post-war Britain was still characterised by conformity to a clearly defined class system and dominated by professional hierarchies. Even though the values of the NHS were derived from socialist principles, the distance between doctors and their patients remained, in most instances, huge. The same was true of the distance between doctors and other healthcare professionals such as nurses, their relative status being reflected in their length of training, remuneration and employment benefits, the nature of the work they did and the career opportunities open to them. Medical power thrived in the NHS and became a barrier to the implementation of change in healthcare practice and management. Additional resources, allocated to those regional teaching hospitals attached to medical schools, served to strengthen the medical profession and created divisions between 'centres of excellence' and hospitals that did not provide medical training. Equality in terms of access to uniformly first-rate services has, therefore, never existed in the NHS, and that situation continues today with the 'postcode lottery', with the service one receives depending on where one lives.

John Thompson was a young finance officer at the Churchill Hospital in Oxford in 1948 when the NHS came into being, and his observations from that period (personal communication, 2007) illuminate the development and present circumstances of the NHS. At the outbreak of war in 1939, he recalls, infections were the principal cause of morbidity and premature death, many having been acquired in hospital. The only drugs available were sulphonamides, bacteriostatic agents that were not anti-biotics. Side effects of sulphonamides were common and included loss of appetite, nausea, vomiting, fever and drowsiness, with risk of kidney failure and death following long-term use (Parish, 1980). During the Second World War, Sir Alexander Fleming discovered penicillin. This powerful new drug was restricted to military personnel and not made available to the public until after the NHS was established. Its amazing properties led doctors to believe that it was a cure for everything. The cost of over- and inappropriate prescribing of the new miracle drug was ignored, however, and unrestricted use led hospitals to run out of penicillin and patients to go without treatment. Although Bevan was aware of the financial pressure being created by penicillin and other new drugs – such as streptomycin, which followed penicillin and was used to combat TB – the situation was allowed to drift. It is ironic that concern over hospital infections, most notably in the form of multi-drug-resistant *Staphylococcus aureus* (MRSA), has once again come to prominence as non-medical prescribing is getting established. The indiscriminate use of anti-biotics coupled with poor hygiene has been blamed.

Within a decade of the inauguration of the NHS, politicians and healthcare planners realised that the experiment was far too ambitious and that the demands being made upon the new service had been completely underestimated (Guillebaud Report, 1956). The nation was far less healthy than had been presumed, and doctors were diagnosing more chronic ill health than had been anticipated. Although the NHS had been promised fast access to services, in reality, people were waiting for long periods to see specialists or for admission to hospital. Treatments such as anti-biotics were not as plentiful as people had been led to believe, and doctors found themselves in the unenviable position of deciding which patients should receive treatment and which should not. Where politicians had assumed that readily available healthcare would quickly redress the effects of war on the nation and that the early identification and treatment of disease would result in Britain re-establishing itself as a superpower, this proved not to be the case. From its inception, the humanistic values underpinning the NHS were insufficient to compensate for ongoing shortages of money and resources, leading to permanent crisis management and rationing of healthcare (Klein *et al.*, 1996).

Nonetheless, during its 60-year existence, the NHS has produced tremendous changes in the health of the nation. Perhaps for the first time medicine can truly claim, on balance, to be doing more good than harm. The *pharmacological revolution* (McNight, 1995) of the last three decades has seen the introduction of new drugs which have made considerable contributions to alleviating suffering. There has been a concomitant escalation in people's expectations that their health problems can be solved with minimal effort on their part. The affluent world is only just beginning to understand that such expectations are unrealistic and that there are limits to what medicine and healthcare can deliver.

Some commentators would not accept that improvements in health can be principally attributed to the NHS. McKeown (1979), formerly Professor of Social Medicine at the University of Birmingham, has argued that medical interventions have contributed relatively little to the health of the nation; far more influential have been higher living standards, improved housing, sanitation and education, and health and safety legislation. In a detailed study of liberal prescribing, Wade (1970), formerly Professor of Therapeutics and Pharmacology at Queen's University, Belfast, and a member of the Medicines Commission, raised concerns about the extent of drug-induced disease in the community. He found that doctors did not take drug-induced side effects seriously and were not concerned to address their prescribing practices.

Current issues with medicines

From a European perspective, Ager (2007) suggests that the pharmaceutical industry has made significant contributions to the treatment of infectious diseases, childhood illnesses, some forms of cancer, nervous disorders, stomach ulcers, asthma, hypertension and diabetes but has made relatively little impact in other areas, such as chronic conditions, migraine, low back pain and diseases of old age. It is expected that current pharmacological research will result in improved treatments in the future for heart disease, HIV/AIDs, Alzheimer's, Parkinson's, arthritis, osteoporosis and cystic fibrosis. In 2005, the pharmaceutical industry in Europe invested over 21 billion Euros in research and development with no certainty of a return on its investment (Ager, 2007).

In the UK, medicines are currently central to healthcare. Approximately £100 billion was spent on medicines in 2006, amounting to 12.2% of the total running costs of the NHS and second only to staff costs (Healthcare Commission, 2007). Few studies have focused on the waste associated with prescribing, but it is thought that around £100 million is spent by government annually on medicines prescribed for patients, *but not taken*. While the figures seem huge, the UK's expenditure on medicines per head of population remains well below that of other countries. The UK comes 13th out of the 15 OECD countries in terms of expenditure on drugs (Garel, 2007).

Approximately half of all prescriptions are taken incorrectly, and some doctors admit they experiences difficulties in relating to some patients (Dean *et al.*, 2002). This is often attributable to poor communication between doctor and patient, with patients being left in ignorance of the benefits and risks of what they are being prescribed (Parish, 1980). High rates of prescribing errors result in iatrogenic harm (Avery *et al.*, 2002; Taxis & Barber, 2003), and Sandars and Esmail 2003 reported that computers recently installed in GP practices fail to warn of potentially fatal prescribing errors. At particular risk are children, pregnant women and older adults. Maidment *et al.* (2006) state that prescribing errors are unacceptably high and approximately 40 000 medication errors occur in the NHS annually, resulting in 2000 (5%) people experiencing moderate to severe harm. Diagnosis of conditions prior to prescribing is often inaccurate (Fairman *et al.*, 1998), and accurate prescribing is difficult for the approximately 17.5 million adults with chronic disease in the UK who present with multiple and complex problems (Humphries & Green, 2002; Mullally, 2004). Patients complain about having a lack of information regarding their medicines and why they are being prescribed (Kass *et al.*, 2000). Furedi (2004) raises philosophical issues around prescribing, questioning whether the current emphasis on medication tends to reinvent people as victims of their own biochemistry, leading them to believe in a 'quick fix' which relieves them of all responsibility for their own health. Cornwell (2006) expresses alarm at the quantity of drugs being prescribed in the Western world for what is perceived to be hyperactivity and at the use of drugs to keep children happy and performing well at school. Vandenbroucke (2004) argues that the first duty of any prescribing clinician is to assess why a drug is being prescribed and to evaluate whether the benefits claimed for the treatments prescribed really exist or whether they are imagined on the part of prescribers and recipients.

Mental health prescribing is characterised by problems surrounding indiscriminate and ill-informed polypharmacy (Paton, 2004) and an unacceptably high incidence of drug errors (Senst *et al.*, 2001). The failure to offer and provide other forms of intervention (Nirodi & Mitchell, 2002) is a situation more prevalent in mental health than any other branch of the health services. Pumariega (2003) notes that there is a tendency to over-medicate mental health clients who live in isolation, although the best outcomes are achieved where pharmacological interventions are closely linked to social and psychological support. Healy (2006) argues that unrealistic expectations of what the drug industry can deliver have created a pool of uncritical prescribers and that the ascendancy of biological theories of mental illness has enhanced the influence of the pharmaceutical industry within mental health care.

Shell (2001) suggests that one in three mental health clients were being medicated inappropriately, and approximately 36% of people with severe mental health problems have been prescribed more than the maximum dose of antipsychotic medication. In a study conducted in a large mental health Trust in England, Paton and Gill-Banham (2003) suggest that majority of errors can be ascribed to failure to apply clinical knowledge or clerical oversight. In 63 cases, 11% of the total, the error could have resulted in a serious incident. This study concludes that prescribing errors are a daily occurrence and that a potentially serious error is likely to occur on a weekly basis in an average mental health Trust. Despite the seriousness of the position, few authors have addressed the problem; those who have have found that there is considerable scope for improving clinical decision making. Denig *et al.* (2002) found that educational strategies for assisting doctors to improve their prescribing decisions were effective in only 50% of cases. Education that focuses primarily on the imparting of knowledge is unlikely to bring about change in practice; however, getting students to critically analyse the processes of their clinical judgement making is more likely to reveal determinants which influence decisions. Perhaps the most obvious explanation for the high rates of mistakes by doctors is the little time devoted to prescribing in medical training and the poor mentoring support junior doctors receive in clinical practice (Talbot, 2004). The lessons from studies such as these are that merely replicating what is currently happening is insufficient and that extending prescribing to other professions must result in more appropriate and beneficial prescribing.

Smith (2002), in an editorial in the *British Medical Journal*, highlights the increasing competition between drug companies as they struggle to retain their share of the market. This has led to ethically questionable practices such as drug trials being conducted in developing countries, where research protocols are less strict than in the West; failure to report unfavourable as well as favourable findings; failure to describe all the characteristics of patients participating in trials and finally rushing drugs onto the market prior to full evaluation. The editorial reserves its sternest criticism for pharmaceutical companies engaged in 'celebrity selling', as illustrated by the recent case of Ricky Williams. A football star with the Miami Dolphins, Williams was adored by the American public. In one of his many television interviews, he stated that he had suffered from 'social anxiety disorder' (shyness), but that since taking paroxetine (Seroxat), the condition had resolved and he had been able to pursue his career. Subsequent probing by the media and the medical profession revealed that the celebrity had been paid an undisclosed sum to mention both the condition and the drug, thereby advertising the drug and suggesting that shy people had a disorder in need of treatment. The manufacturers, GlaxoSmithKline, subsequently amassed profits in excess of US $2.7 billion in 1 year from the sale of paroxetine. The drug has been a subject of the BBC investigative journalism programme *Panorama* (29 January 2007) and has been withdrawn in the UK for patients under the age of 18 because of its alleged links with suicide.

Media investigation has generated scepticism about the honesty of the pharmaceutical industry in marketing its products. Doctors are realising that their profession may have overestimated the benefits of medication by overlooking the fact that compliant patients might tell them that their conditions have improved as a result of medication when in fact they feel no different or worse (Paton & Gill-Banham, 2003). The National Institute for Clinical Excellence (NICE) now aims to subject pharmacological interventions to more intense scrutiny than has been the case in the past (Department of Health [DoH], 2006a), although some critics have suggested that the remit of NICE is not to recommend the best medicines but the *cheapest* (Mandelstam, 2006). However, with the extension of prescribing rights to disciplines other than medicine and the traditional hierarchy within healthcare established in the eighteenth and nineteenth centuries rapidly disappearing, prescribing is surely going to be evaluated far more rigorously.

Appleyard (2007) sees political preoccupation with heath and healthcare services as having both intended and unintended consequences. By promising improved services and a wider range of choices, more treatments and better care, people's expectations are raised beyond what can realistically be met. Media coverage of the latest developments in medicine and pharmaceuticals leads the public to believe that these advances are instantly available to anyone who wants them and that healthcare services can enable people to live longer, happier and more fulfilled lives. Mankind, Appleyard (2007) argues, has always wanted to prolong its sojourn on earth and will believe in anything that appears to hold out the prospect of cheating death, be it throwing bones or the latest technology. In reality, the fact that medicines are manufactured does not mean they are available for everyone or appropriate for every condition, as Clark (2007), a former nurse and a cancer sufferer, discovered when she was refused Herceptin on the grounds that it was not appropriate for her cancer. She argued that while it might not be the most appropriate drug, it was the best available at the time, and denying her access to it contravened the NHS Plan (DoH 2006b). She and other similar patients were subsequently prescribed the drug when the then Secretary of Health over-ruled the decision of various PCTs to withhold it.

A similar situation arose with Aricept, a drug used in the treatment of Alzheimer's disease. Doctors were advised not to prescribe it on the grounds of its questionable effectiveness, but carers and relatives claimed that it was being refused simply because of the cost and that there was no comparable drug on the market. Controversy also arose about Aimspro, marketed as a wonder drug for the treatment of the UK's 85,000 multiple sclerosis sufferers. Although the drug was originally allowed to be sold under 'special licence', the Medicines and Healthcare Products Regulatory Agency (MHRA) had second thoughts after the 'elephant man' drugs trial at Northwick Park Hospital in 2006, which left six healthy young men critically ill. The company behind the drug, Daval International, was accused of a lack of transparency regarding the trialling of the drug and the claims made on its behalf (Gillard *et al.*, 2006). NICE argues that medicines must provide value for money, otherwise there is no justification for public monies to be spent on them. This position resonates with that of Medawar (1986), who advised that the medical profession should not be seeking new drugs but endeavouring to make the best of the ones already available.

In 2006, sales of pharmaceuticals reached $602 billion worldwide. The industry is currently enjoying a growth rate of 7% per annum. In a study of the major pharmaceutical companies (Consumers International, 2006), a number of ethical issues were highlighted:

- Not all companies were transparent about their marketing practices.
- Not all companies provided full information about research trials.
- As companies cannot sell directly to clients, some targeted patient groups, medical students and pharmacists to market their products.
- Health information leaflets, which purported to be neutral, could be heavily weighted towards products.
- Self-regulation in the industry is weak and generally inadequate to protect consumers from potentially misleading information.

Drug companies are now coming under pressure from many directions. There is increased interest in and sales of complementary medicines, which can be accessed outside the NHS through the Internet, supermarkets and other high street outlets. The food industry has also responded to an increasingly health-aware public by developing dietary supplements, reducing sugar and fat in its products and offering healthy living advice. The Office of Fair Trading's recent report (2007) on a study undertaken to assess whether the NHS got value for money from the drug companies concluded that the £8 billion worth of medicines bought by the NHS did not represent good value for money. Drug companies were reported as charging excessively for medicines prescribed for high cholesterol, high blood pressure and stomach problems. Moynihan *et al.* (2002) commented wryly that there now appears to be 'an ill for every pill' and questioned the philosophy of making excessive amounts of drugs available. Some of the drugs purchased by the NHS were found to be 500 times more expensive than alternative products for the same conditions. The Office of Fair Trading did not lay the blame for this situation at the door of the drug companies but declared that NHS purchasers were neither as informed nor as rigorous as they should be. Drugs should be assessed on three criteria:

- Are they reasonably priced?
- Are there discernible benefits to patients?
- Does the price allow the company to carry out further research?

Drug companies have a very short period of time, usually about 2 years, in which to recoup their outlay on a new drug. Once the drug comes off patent, any company can market it, and the cost goes down. When Viagra, a drug manufactured by Pfizer for erectile dysfunction, came off patent, it was manufactured by Eli Lilly, a rival company, and went on sale in Boots on St Valentine's Day 2007 at a much reduced cost (Goodman & Templeton, 2007).

The pharmaceutical industry finds itself further challenged by the rise of 'Internet pharmacies' and 'cyber-doctoring'. It is estimated that 2300 sites exist worldwide where prescription-only drugs are sold directly to the consumer. The most frequently bought drugs are sleeping pills, anti-depressants, painkillers, Viagra and Valium. These unregulated sources of medicines expose patients to serious health risks and addiction. Poorly or incorrectly labelled medicines are sent out that are substandard and in some cases lethal. In Britain the National Audit Office has estimated that at least 600 000 people have used the Internet to buy prescription drugs and in many instances do not inform their GPs that they are taking them (Coralli, 2006). While a post-modern approach to health-care suggests that individuals should take responsibility for their own health, self-medication is fraught with problems and dangers (Bunton & Burows, 1995).

The essence of good prescribing, states Moerman (2002), is that the prescriber adopt the role of collaborator and guide rather than expert giving directives to the patient. Placebo studies have yielded important insights into the importance of taking the patient's own understanding of his on her condition into account. How a patient thinks about health, illness and treatment may determine the outcome of treatment. Beecher (1961) found that 35% of improvement could be attributed to the placebo effect or the belief that patients had in their treatment. Hence, patient education, information-giving and motivational interviewing should be an essential part of modern prescribing. Pilgrim and Bentall (1999) argue that the history of medicine is largely the history of the placebo effect; when patients have improved, it has been because of their belief in the treatment rather than the efficacy of the treatment. The illness may be ongoing, but the patient's behaviour indicates improved health.

Lundkvist *et al.* (2002) claim that it is futile to try to explain why a patient gets better without knowing the natural course of the illness and the likelihood of eventual recovery. Depending on the characteristics of the illness and the patient, some or most patients will recover even without treatment. For example, almost everyone can recover from the common cold without taking any medicines. It is therefore important to identify recovery as a part of the natural course of the condition and differentiate it from the effect of placebo and treatment (Kinnersley *et al.*, 1999).

In 1994, the Health Education Authority (HEA) identified that unsupported medical treatments were unlikely to be successful:

> The best results are attained when treatments are accompanied by actions on a number of other fronts including legislation, policies, environmental measures and the promotion of healthy lifestyles. These other activities and services are collectively referred to as 'health promotion'. Health promotion is the responsibility of a wide range of agencies at all levels, e.g. social care, local government, workplaces, commerce and voluntary groups. Any successful strategy to improve health will therefore be based on coordinated action through agencies working together in 'alliances for health'. (page 45)

The HEA had earlier stated that:

> Health is not a state or a fact; it is more like an idea or an opinion, and our views of health are based on our values and our experiences. Although there are more ways than subjective ones of looking at health, they are important. (page 3)

Naidoo and Wills (2000) claim that since the introduction of the NHS, it has become increasingly apparent that the biomedical model is less than convincing in understanding and seeking to cure such recalcitrant problems as cancer, heart disease, chronic pain, violent anti-social behaviour and some forms of drug abuse. Ewles and Simnett (1999) contend that good health behaviours are far more successful in promoting wellness than medicines. Such habits include sleeping 7 to 8 hours a night, being less than 10% overweight, eating breakfast every day, not eating between meals, taking regular exercise, not smoking, and consuming alcohol sensibly. Katz and Peberdy (1997) see healthcare as shifting towards the social sciences, where behavioural and medical scientists collaborate. Health outcomes, they argue, are better where the locus of control is not with the professional but with the patient, who is supported to take responsibility for his or her own health.

Leibovici and Lievre (2002) consider that science in general, and medical science in particular, is deliberately debated in a way that makes it beyond the reach of ordinary people. When doctors and scientists fail to communicate with the public and to clarify the values underpinning their work, they expose themselves to accusations of elitism and self-interest. Healthcare knowledge and its dissemination may be in urgent need of democratisation. Medical practitioners exercise enormous power and control over people's lives, power that has been given to them by their patients, who choose to believe that doctors can protect them from the ravages of old age, pain and disability. Doctors may be tempted to overreach themselves when the public insists on *a cheap magic charm to prevent, and a cheap pill or potion to cure all diseases* (Shaw, 1946).

However, there are many instances in which doctors are called upon to assist people for whose conditions there is no specific treatment and when the options available to them are no better than what people could do for themselves. As Shaw (1946) commented in *The Doctor's Dilemma* (1946):

Make it compulsory for a doctor using a brass plate to have inscribed on it, in addition to the letters indicating his qualifications, the words, *Remember that I am mortal.*

Modernising healthcare

The introduction of the internal market in healthcare during the Thatcher governments of the 1980s was an attempt to curtail spiralling costs, but it achieved only modest results. Following the landslide victory of the Labour Government in 1997, Tony Blair, then prime minister, intimated that the Labour Party was the natural party to put right the problems within the NHS; after all, it was a Labour Government creation (Kirklin & Richardson, 2001). The rationale for modernisation took into account new medical technologies, an aging population, escalating public expectations and an outdated NHS management style. The old-fashioned paternalism that characterised healthcare was no longer acceptable to patients, who wanted to be treated more as customers than guinea pigs. In any case, immediate radical overhaul of the NHS was needed in order to avert a financial crisis that threatened to destroy it. Policy makers and politicians set about a 'root and branch' reform that would have far-reaching consequences for providers of healthcare, patients and the public at large. A plethora of policy documents, unprecedented in the history of healthcare, set out to transform all aspects of the NHS, bringing in new services, roles, pay scales and methods of training. The rate at which policies were published far exceeded the ability of NHS personnel to keep pace.

The Modernisation Agency was formed in 2001 with the aim of coordinating policies, facilitating change and accelerating the speed with which it could be achieved. In July 2005, it was replaced by the NHS Institute for Innovation and Improvement, which adhered largely to the same agenda but signalled that there was considerably more scope for innovation. Change agents were constantly reminded that they must take into account the local context of healthcare provision so that the centrally controlled NHS that had existed for almost half a century could be replaced by one responsive to individual and local needs. Good will alone, however, has proved insufficient to bring about change everywhere; in some places, change has been welcomed, but in others the attempt to modernise has been met with negativity and led to frustration (DoH, 2006). Theorists concur that change is best assimilated when it is phased in and all those expected to bring about change are involved in what is happening from the beginning (Neal & Biberman, 2004; Lotte *et al.*, 2006). Too rapid a flow of policy documents can result in organisations' failing to address problems systematically. Kivimaki *et al.* (1998) found that over-exposure to change in organisations can have

adverse effects on the workforce, particularly a workforce that is poorly prepared and supported.

Non-medical prescribing was a major innovation introduced into the NHS
towards the end of the twentieth century. Its primary aim was to provide patients
with faster access to medicines; subsidiary aims included reducing waiting lists
and creating a more flexible and responsive workforce. This meant that for the
first time in the UK, at least some of those who traditionally administered prescribed medicines now had the responsibility of prescribing them as well. Few
directions were given initially as to how exactly non-medical prescribing was to
be implemented; this evolved as the process got under way. Today, what is happening in any particular geographical area or field of practice depends on who is
delivering the service. The first group to embrace non-medical prescribing was
the nursing profession. Nurses already had close connections with prescribing
and were used to explaining medicines to patients and supporting them during
their treatment. Nurses were soon followed by pharmacists, physiotherapists,
radiographers and podiatrists. A close observation of the introduction of nurse
prescribing permits the implementation to be observed from the perspective of
nurses themselves and the experiences they encountered.

Non-doctor prescribing in the UK

Ever since the Medical Registration Act of 1858, doctors have been invested with
powers to diagnose, prescribe and take responsibility for the overall management
of patients. Medical dominance was achieved in the absence of scientific evidence
that what doctors did was useful, and largely as a result of the social standing of
doctors. While nurses were the mainstay of hospitals, they were bound by the
rules of the institution and the dictates of medical personnel.

It is tempting to attribute any significant new development to the influence of
a few visionary and strong-minded people or to a few well-documented events,
when in reality events and individuals simply give expression to a zeitgeist that
has been gradually developing. Nonetheless, there are 'movers and shakers' and,
in the case of non-medical prescribing, one of these was Baroness Julia Cumberlege. At a conference in Staffordshire in 2003, she revealed that she had become
involved in non-medical prescribing quite serendipitously (Cumberlege, 2003).
In 1982, she was appointed to chair the Brighton Health Authority and shortly
after was invited by the Minister of Health, Kenneth Clarke, to undertake a review
of community nursing. One of the principal recommendations arising from her
review was that nurse prescribing should be introduced in order to improve the
quality of care available in the community. Cumberlege was aware that nurse
prescribing had been successfully established in the United States for at least
two decades and believed that it could be equally successful in Britain. She felt
that nursing had made substantial professional progress over the previous two

decades, with the shift from an NHS-based training to a university-based one. Following her report, Dr. June Crown, a community physician, was asked to chair an advisory group. It soon became obvious that not all nurses were well disposed towards the proposal; many were ensconced in traditional ways of working and were unwilling to move on. However, Trevor Clay, General Secretary of the Royal College of Nursing, and some pharmacists had been strong supporters of non-medical prescribing and the benefits it could yield for patients. Some doctors were also strongly opposed on the grounds that this had been traditionally the province of doctors, that nurses had insufficient training in pharmacology and that there were no additional resources to implement non-medical prescribing. It took 17 years to implement nurse prescribing across the country. The first community Trust where all district nurses qualified as prescribers was Bolton, in the northwest of England.

Reflecting on what had been achieved with respect to non-medical prescribing in the UK, Crown (2006) noted that the fact that over 30 000 district nurses and health visitors, over 8000 other nurses, including 600 mental health nurses, and over 1000 pharmacists were registered as prescribers was evidence that the initiative had well and truly taken off. A major reason for developing nurse prescribing had been to recognise both the work that nurses were doing and what they were capable of. By November 2006, 13 physiotherapists and 8 chiropodist/podiatrists were also registered to prescribe.

Although the number of non-medical prescribers is continually increasing, their contribution to prescribing in primary care remains relatively small. During 2005, nurses prescribed medicines to the value of £61 million, or 0.8% of the £7823 million spent by GPs on prescribing (National Prescribing Centre, 2006). This figure may conceal the fact that nurses are prescribing a wide range of medicines but less expensive ones than those prescribed by doctors.

Reflecting on the course of non-medical prescribing, Crown made the following observations at the 6th Non-Medical Prescribing Conference in Stafford in 2006:

- The aim of introducing non-doctor prescribing was to improve health outcomes for patients. It was seen as a waste of resources when nurses were seeing patients, assessing them, deciding what they needed and then having to find a junior doctor, not nearly as experienced and knowledgeable as they were, to sign a prescription. Nurse prescribing was never intended to address the problem of too few doctors. The solution to the problem of too few doctors was seen as more doctors, not nurse prescribers.
- In the early days of non-medical prescribing, nurses were pushed through the training whether they wanted to prescribe or not. This proved counterproductive in that reluctant nurses, once qualified, simply did not prescribe. Since then, nurses have gone forward to train providing (a) they want to and (b) it is clear that prescribing will make a difference to their clinical practice and (c) to the organisation in which they are working.

- The implementation of nurse prescribing highlighted deeply rooted conservatism in the NHS and the nursing profession. Once the legislation for non-medical prescribing was in place, it took nearly 10 years before the scheme was rolled out nationally.
- Non-medical extended prescribing makes a significant difference to people with long-standing conditions. Patients with conditions that follow an uneven course benefit from having their medication checked regularly. Signs of deterioration are detected earlier.
- In mental health services, specialist nurses are well placed to play a major part in supervising the care of patients with whom they often build up strong helping relationships.
- The mentoring of trainee mental health nurse prescribers is likely to change in the next few years. Consultant psychiatrists may no longer be considered the best people to act as mentors. General practitioners may become more involved, and in due course, interdisciplinary supervision groups could be established comprising nurses, physiotherapists and pharmacists. This will facilitate a new outlook on prescribing, different from the medical model.
- Non-medical prescribing underlines how important it is for health professionals to work within their competencies and scope of practice. The Shipman Report made it clear to health professionals that they have a responsibility to keep an eye on colleagues' practice and, if deficient, to take action.

Nursing and the current NHS context

It is undoubtedly the case that nurses numerically far exceed any other professional group with respect to non-medical prescribing, but that does not mean that what they do is effective, providing better access to care and treatment and meeting the needs of patients who have been poorly served in the past. However, it must be borne in mind that the rise of non-medical prescribing is only one dimension of a range of other innovations that have sought to provide faster access to care and services for service users and their carers, offer more varied choice to patients, provide better opportunities for the utilisation of non-medical skills and knowledge and make better use of resources. The growing expectations of what can actually be delivered by non-medical prescribing and the constant reassurances given by government that all healthcare expectations can be met must give rise to concern. Much of the recent innovation introduced has been imposed on Trusts in the form of outcomes; little has been generated as a result of consultations with the public. As has been hinted at in this chapter, the tendency on the part of all governments to promise more in terms of health than the country can actually afford still continues. It is interesting that the optimism of Cumberlege and Crown, both non-nurses, paid scant attention to the reality of nursing (e.g. recruitment and retention, pay and career prospects). The recent Modernising Nursing Careers (DoH, 2006a) outlined the biggest health problems in England today. It acknowledges that after 50 years of the NHS, healthcare is not distributed equally and inequalities continue to be a major challenge. People have more access to information than ever before and expect to be treated as partners. The cost of new treatments and new information systems means greater focus on value for money. In addition to society becoming more complex, the key changes impacting on the delivery of health services are the following facts:

- The number of people aged over 85 years is projected to rise by nearly 75% by 2025.
- Over 15 million people in the UK have a long-term condition, and as the number of older people increases, this figure is also likely to increase by approximately 23%
- Obesity rates have doubled in the last 10 years, potentially leading to more strokes, heart attacks and type 2 diabetes. It is estimated that 1 in 4 people will be obese by 2010.
- Infant mortality rates vary from 1.6 per 1000 live births in Eastleigh to 9.8 per 1000 live births in Birmingham.
- Smoking is still the greatest cause of illness and premature death in the UK, killing at least 86 500 annually and accounting for a third of all cancers and a seventh of all cardiovascular disease.

Several studies carried out by nurses seem to indicate that the introduction of nurse prescribing has gone some way in addressing these and other problems and has met with approval from patients (Luker, 1997; Mundinger *et al.*, 2000; Hemingway, 2004; Courtnay *et al.*, 2005; Clegg, *et al.*, 2006). The early work of Mundinger (2002) demonstrated that nurse prescribers were especially effective in managing 'first contact' patients in rural and underserved areas, where few doctors elected to work. Taking a comprehensive view of healthcare in the United States, Running (2006) claimed that healthcare resources were in crisis and were not available to an ever-growing number of people with complex needs. She warned that merely extending the roles of nurses and creating new ones would have little impact on the health outcomes of the nation if appropriate resources were not available to support them. Her study supported the findings of Mundinger (2002), but she also found that nurses, who were more effective than doctors in prescribing for certain patients, combined a medical-based approach with a health-belief model that includes teaching and motivation to move clients towards better health. Hence, it was the approach adopted by the nurse rather than the efficacy of the medicines prescribed that accounted for most of the health gain. Both of these authors argue that the reorganisation of healthcare in the United States is due largely to how healthcare will be funded in the future and not to discovering how services could be improved. Evidence exists that some nurses, on completion of their prescribing courses, do not return to the service they worked in prior to embarking on the course because they would not be able to practice in the way they had expected; instead, they seek out services where their skills are appreciated (Fontana *et al.*, 2000). The obvious implication is that services and service managers need to be clear about the value of the role, otherwise highly motivated staff could move elsewhere.

A growing number of authors in the UK are beginning to question the current position of nursing and what nurses are being asked to do. Shields and Watson (2007) argue that nursing is being assassinated in a misguided attempt at cost cutting, which will result in an electoral backlash and the early deaths of patients from unskilled and inadequate care. They concur with the arguments advanced by Clay (1987) that educating nurses to the highest possible standards is the best means of improving the quality of health and is cost-effective. They point out that approximately 50% of the current nursing workforce is due to retire within the next decade, that less than 4% of those qualified in 2005–2006 were graduates and that nursing is being increasingly taught by lecturers who have little time for self-development or involvement in practice. The dumbing down of education is taking place at a time when there is a burgeoning increase in technology used in healthcare, which requires a depth of knowledge of physics, chemistry, biology and genomics. Furthermore, it seems curious that when Ireland has moved towards a graduate nursing profession and Wales and Scotland are planning to do so, England has no such plans. Engineering healthcare so that nurses and others take on what was previously doctors' work may have initial attractions, but in the long term it could seriously undermine the whole edifice of healthcare.

Godin (1996) considers that initiatives that purport to advance nursing, such as nurse prescribing, are futile attempts by some nurses to gain autonomy over some aspects of healthcare work. Nursing, he argues, is dominated by a general nursing elite who have orchestrated recent reforms towards genericism and homogeneity, thus marginalising specialist groups such as mental health and learning disability nurses. He focuses particularly on the work of some CPNs who have no desire to be associated with nurse prescribing and furthermore do not see any necessity for doctors to be involved with people whose problems are primarily social and cognitive. These nurses wish to distance themselves from medicines, particularly depot injections, in favour of therapeutic interventions that require social, cognitive and spiritual skills, which they believe is the essence of nursing. He suggests that many mental health and learning disability teams will find it difficult to sustain non-medical prescribing because these teams lack equality, integration and a stable division of labour. Instead, they have become arenas in which occupational groups strive for dominance, vie with each other for privileges and remuneration and seek ways of gaining access to clients who pose the least challenge. Holmes (2006) points to several other caring groups who feel under siege and whose plight is being ignored by government and their immediate employers (e.g. health visitors, older adult nurses, midwives and mental health nurses). Older people with health and social care needs also frequently complain that they are disadvantaged with respect to the resources that are available to them. The traditional situation of nursing is under threat, he argues, owing to poor recruitment and retention, indifferent education and training opportunities, low job satisfaction and poor career prospects. These authors conclude that developments such as nurse prescribing only serve to cover up the underlying problems in healthcare and will eventually serve to fragment the profession, while at the same time undermining medicine.

It is not an accident that the emergence of a primary care–led NHS has coincided with a movement towards healthy living. 'Healthism', as it is frequently referred to, has now become a central tenet of consumer culture fuelled by media messages regarding youth and fitness based on healthy eating, alternative therapies, membership of sports and health clubs, cosmetic surgery and psychoanalysis (Burrows *et al.*, 1995). The emphasis on a health-promoting lifestyle represents a new approach to healthcare, distinctly different from that of traditional medicine which stepped in once illness had declared itself and in many instances removed the sufferer from his or her familiar context. Preventive, non-institutional, participative approaches to healthcare contrast with traditional approaches to sickness, which were curative and institutionally based (Bunton & Burrows, 1995). So where does non-medical prescribing sit? And where are the initial practitioners based? And are they abiding by the old curative approach or embracing the newly emerging health-promotion one?

Although the policies are explicit about what non-medical prescribing could achieve and there are some point-prevalence studies stating what is being achieved, there is as yet no cohort study which seeks to observe non-medical prescribing through the eyes and experiences of those engaged in it. It is an examination of this reality on which the following chapters focus.

REFERENCES

Ager, B. (2007) The research-based pharmaceutical industry – a key actor for a healthy Europe. In: *The Official Hope Reference Book*. London: Camden Publishing Limited.

Appleyard, B. (2007) *How to Live Forever or Die Trying: On the New Morality*. London: Simon & Schuster.

Avery, A., Sheikh, A., Hurwitz, B., Smeaton, L., Chen-Yen, F., Howard, R. (2002) Safer medicines management in primary care. *British Journal of General Practice*, **52**, 517–22.

Bates, D. W., Cullen, D. J., Laird, N. *et al.* (1995) Incidence of adverse drug events and potential adverse drug events: implications for prevention. *Journal of the American Medical Association*, **274**, 29–34.

Beecher, H. K. (1961) Surgery as placebo: a quantative study of bias. *Journal of the American Medical Association*, **296**, 1102–7.

Black, N. (2006) *Walking London's Medical History*. London: The Royal Society of Medicine Press Ltd.

Bunton, R. & Burrows, R. (1995) Consumption and health in the 'epidemiological' clinic of late modern medicine. In: S. Nettleton & R. Burrows (eds) *The Sociology of Health Promotion*. London: Routledge.

Burrows, R., Nettleton, S. & Bunton, R. (1995) Health risk and consumption under late modernism, In: S. Nettleton & R. Burrows (eds) *The Sociology of Health Promotion*. London: Routledge.

Campbell, D. (1926) *Arabian Medicine and Its Influence in the Middle Ages*. New York: J. B. Lippincott Company.

Clark, B. (2007) *The Fight of My Life*. London: Simon & Schuster.

Consumers International (2006) *Branding the Cure. A Consumer Perspective on Corporate Social Responsibility, Drug Promotion and the Pharmaceutical Industry in Europe*. London: Consumers International.

Clay, T. (1987) *Nurses: Power and Politics*. London: Heinemann Nursing.

Clegg, A., Meades, R. & Broderick, W. (2006) Reflections on nurse independent prescribing in hospital settings. *Nursing Standard*, **21**, 35–7.

Coralli, C. (2006) Effective case presentations – an important clinical skill for nurse practitioners. *Journal of American Academy of Nurse Practitioners*, **18**(5), 216–21.

Cornwell, J. (2006) Chemical kids, *The Sunday Times Magazine*, 12 November, pp. 16–24.

Courtnay, M., Young, A. & Dunn, N. (2005) *An Evaluation of Extended Formulary Independent Nurse Prescribing*. Executive summary of the final report. Policy Research Programme at the Department of Health and the University of Southampton. London: Department of Health.

Crown, J. (2006) *Reflections on the Introduction of Nurse Prescribing – What Has Been Achieved. Hoar Cross Hall Conference Centre*. South Staffordshire NHS Foundation Trust.

Cumberlege, J. (2003) A triumph of sense over tradition: the development of nurse prescribing. *Nurse Prescribing*, **1**, 10–14.

Cumberlege, J. (2003) *Keynote Address, 'Dicing with My Mental Health'*. South Staffordshire Healthcare NHS Trust.

Dean, B., Schachter, M., Vincent, C. & Barber, N. (2002) Causes of prescribing errors in hospital inpatients: a prospective study. *The Lancet*, **359**, 1373–8.

Denig, P., Wahlstrom, R., & Chaput de Saintonge, M. (2002) The value of clinical judgement analysis for improving the quality of doctors' prescribing decisions. *Medical Education*, **36**, 770–8.

Department of Health (2006a) *Modernising Nursing Careers*. London: The Stationery Office.

Department of Health (2006b) *Improving Patients' Access to Medicines: A Guide to Implementing Nurse and Pharmacist Independent Prescribing within the NHS in England*. London: Department of Health.

Ewles, L. & Simnett, I. (1999) *Promoting Health: A Practical Guide*, 4th edn. Edinburgh: Bailliere Tindall.

Fairman, K., Drevets W., Kreisman, J. & Teitbaum, F. (1998) Course of antidepressant treatment drug type, and prescriber speciality. *Psychiatric Services*, **49**, 1180–6.

Fontana, S., Devine, E. C. & Kelber, S. K. (2000) Nurse practitioner prescriber student prescription patterns. *Journal of the American Academy of Nurse Practitioners*, **12**, 3–10.

Furedi, F. (2004) *Therapy Culture*. London: Routledge.

Gardiner, A. H. (1938) The house of life. *Journal of Egyptian Archaeology*, **24**, 157–79.

Garel, P. (2007) Tackling the important issues in European healthcare. In: *The Official Hope Reference Book*. London: Camden Publishing Limited.

Gillard, M., Calvert, J. & Walsh, G. (2006) Criminal probe into MS 'wonder drug'. London: *The Sunday Times*, 26 November, p. 5.

Guillebaud Report (1956) *Report of the Committee of Inquiry into the Cost of the National Health Service*. London: HMSO.

Godin, P. (1996) The development of community psychiatric nursing; a professional project. *Journal of Advanced Nursing*, **23**, 925–34.

Goodman, M. & Templeton, S. K. (2007) Boots puts Viagra on sale for Valentine's Day. London: *The Sunday Times*, p. 7.

Healy, D. (2006) The antidepressant tale: figures signifying nothing? *Advances in Psychiatric Treatment*, **12**, 320–7.

Health Education Authority (1993) *Delivering Health to the Nation*. London: Health Education Authority.

Healthcare Commission (2007) *Talking about Medicines*. London: Healthcare Commission.

Hemingway, S. (2004) The mental health nurse's perspective on implementing nurse prescribing. *Nurse Prescribing*, **2** (1), 37–44.

Holmes, C. A. (2006) The slow death of psychiatric nursing: what next. *Journal of Psychiatric and Mental Health Nursing*, **13**, 401–15.

Hudson, R. P. (1983) *Disease and Its Control: The Shaping of Modern Thought*. Westport, Connecticut: Greenwood Press.

Humphries, J. L., & Green, J. (eds) (2002) *Nurse Prescribing*, 2nd edn. Suffolk, UK: Palgrave Publishers.

Inglis, B. (1981) *The Diseases of Civilisation*. London: Paladin.

Kass, M. J., Dehn, D., & Dahl, D. *et al.* (2000) A view of prescriptive collaboration: perspectives of psychiatric mental health clinical nurse specialists and psychiatrists. *Archives of Psychiatric Nursing*, **14**, 222–34.

Katz, J. & Peberdy, A. (eds) (1997) *Promoting Health: Knowledge and Practice*. Basingstoke, UK: Macmillan and Open University.

Kinnersley, P., Stott, N., Peters, T. J. & Harvey, I. (1999) The patient-centeredness of consultations and outcomes in primary care. *British Journal of General Practice*, **49**, 711–16.

Kirklin, D. & Richardson, R. (2001) *Medical Humanities*. London: Royal College of Physicians.

Kivimaki, M., Vahtera, H., Koskenvuo, M., Uutela, U. & Pentti, A. (1998) *Psychological Medicine*, **28**, 903–13.

Klein, R., Day, P. & Redmayne, S. (1996) *Managing Scarcity*. Buckingham, UK: Open University Press.

Kynaston, D. (2007) *Austerity Britain 1945–51*. London: Bloomsbury.

Leibovici, L. & Lievre, M. (2002) Medicalisation: peering from the inside medicine. *British Medical Journal*, **324**, 866.

Lotte, S., Lewis, M. & Ingram, A. (2006) The social construction of organisational change paradoxes. *Journal of Organisational Change*, **19**, 502–6.

Luker, K. (1997) *Evaluation of Nurse Prescribing. Final Report.* Liverpool: University of Liverpool and University of York.

Lundkvist, J., Akerlind, I., Borgquist, L. & Molstad, S. (2002) The more time spent on listening, the less time spent on prescribing antibiotics in general practice. *Family Practice*, **19**, 638–40.

Maidment, I., Lelliott, P. & Paton, C. (2006) A systematic review of medication errors in mental healthcare. *Quality & Safety in Healthcare*, **15**, 409–13.

Mandelstam, M. (2006) *Betraying the NHS: Health Abandoned.* London: Jessica Kingsley.

McKeown, T. (1979) *The Role of Medicine; Dream, Mirage or Nemesis?* Oxford, UK: Oxford University Press.

McNight, J. (1995) *The Careless Society.* New York: Basic Books.

Medawar, C. (1986) The Spirit of Nairobi. Paper presented at the International Workshop at the Nordic School of Public Health, Gothenberg, Sweden, June 1986, p. 3.

Moerman, D. E. (2002) *Meaning, Medicine and the Placebo Effect.* Cambridge, UK: Cambridge University Press.

Moynihan, R., Heath, I. & Henry, D. (2002) Selling sickness: the pharmacological industry and disease mongering. *British Medical Journal*, **886**, 891.

Mullally, S. (2004) The 6th National Conference for the Association for Nurse Prescribing, 12–13 February, Manchester, UK.

Mundinger, M. O. (2002) Twenty-first century primary care: new partnerships between nurses and doctors, *Academic Medicine*, **77**, 776–80.

Mundinger, M. O., Kane, R. L., Lenz, E. R., Totten, A. M. & Tsai, W. Y. (2000) Primary care outcomes in patients treated by nurse practitioners or physicians: a randomised controlled trial. *Journal of the American Medical Association*, **283**, 59–68.

National Prescribing Centre (2006) *Hospital Medicines Management Collaborative – End of Programme Report 2006.* Liverpool: National Prescribing Centre.

Naidoo, J. & Wills, J. (2000) *Health Promotion – Foundations for Practice*, 2nd edn. London: Bailliere Tindall and Royal College of Nursing.

Neal, J. & Biberman, J. (2004) Research that matters: helping organisations integrate spiritual values and practices. *Journal of Organisational Change Management*, **17**, 10–18.

Nirodi, P. & Mitchell, A. (2002) The quality of psychotropic drug prescribing in patients in psychiatric units for the elderly. *Aging and Mental Health*, **6**, 191–6.

Nunn, J, F. (1996) *Ancient Egyptian Medicine.* London: The British Museum Press.

Office of Fair Trading (2007) Pharmaceutical price regulation scheme Press release 20 Feb. 2007. http://www.oft.gov.uk/advice_and_ resources/resource_base/market-studies/price-regulation (accessed 14 April 2007).

Olie, J. P. & Loo, H. (1999) New drug therapies. In: H. Freeman (ed), *A Century of Psychiatry.* London: Mosby-Wolfe.

Panorama, 'Secrets of the drug trials.' BBC Programme, broadcast 29 January, 2007.

Parish, P. (1980) *Medicines, A Guide for Everybody.* London: Penguin Books.

Paton, C. & Gill-Banham, S. (2003) Prescribing errors in psychiatry. *Psychiatric Bulletin*, **27**, 208–10.

Paton, C., Lelliott, P., Harrington, M. & Okcha, C. (2003) Patterns of antipsychotic prescribing for hospital inpatients. *Journal of Psychopharmacology*, **17**, 223–39.

Paton, N. (2004) Patients behaving badly. *Nursing Times*, **100**(45), 26–7.

Pilgrim, D. & Bentall, R. (1999) The medicalisation of misery: a critical realist analysis of the concept of depression. *Journal of Mental Health*, **8**, 261–74.

Porter, R. (1997) *The Greatest Benefit to Mankind*. London: HarperCollins.

Porter, R. (2004) *The Enlightenment*. London: Palgrave.

Pumariega, A. (2003) Trends and shifting ecologies. *Child and Adolescent Psychiatric Clinics of North America*, **12**, 779–93.

Rawcliffe, C. (1999) *Medicine for the Soul*. Stroud, UK: Sutton Publishing.

Running, A. (2006) Prescriptive patterns of nurse practitioners and physicians. *Journal of the American Academy of Nurse Practitioners*, **18**, 228–33.

Sandars, J. & Esmail, A. (2003) The frequency and nature of medical errors in primary care: understanding the diversity across studies. *Family Practice*, **20**, 231–6.

Saur, C. D. & Ford, S. M. (1995) Quality, cost-effective psychiatric treatment: a CNS-MD collaborative practice model. *Archives of Psychiatric Nursing*, **9**(6), 332–7.

Seacole, M. (1990) *Wonderful Adventures of Mrs. Seacole in Many Lands*. Oxford: Oxford University Press.

Shaw, B. (1946) *The Doctor's Dilemma*. Harmondsworth, UK: Penguin.

Shell, R. C. (2001) Antidepressant prescribing practices of nurse practitioners. *The Nurse Practitioner*, **26**, 42–47.

Shields, L. & Watson, R. (2007) The demise of nursing in the United Kingdom: a warning for medicine. *Journal of the Royal Society of Medicine*, **100**, 70–4.

Smith, R. (2002) Too much medicine, editorial. *British Medical Journal*, **324**, 859–60.

Sonnedecker, G. (1976) *History of Pharmacy*. Philadelphia: J. B. Lippincott Company.

Senst, B., Achusim, L., Genest, R. & Ford, C. (2001) Practical approach to determining costs of frequency and adverse drug events in a health care network. *American Journal of Health System Pharmacy*, **58**, 1126–32.

Swinford, S. (2006) Scientists quit in dyslexia 'cure' row. *The Sunday Times*, 26 November, page 9.

Strouhal, E. (1992) *Life in Ancient Egypt*. Norman: University of Oklahoma Press.

Talbot, M. (2004) Good wine may need to mature: a critique of accelerated higher specialist training. Evidence from cognitive neuroscience. *Medical Education*, **38**, 399–402.

Taxis, K. & Barber, N. (2003) Causes of intravenous medication errors: an ethnographic study. *Quality and Safety in Health Care*, **12**, 343–7.

Vandenbroucke, J. P. (2004) Benefits and harms of drug treatments, editorial. *British Medical Journal*, **329**, 2–3.

Wade, O. L. (1970) *Adverse Reactions to Drugs*. London: Penguin.

Wear, A. (ed) (1992) *Medicine in Society: Historical Essays*. Cambridge, UK: Cambridge University Press.

Webster, C. (1988) *The Health Service Since the War*, vol 1, *The NHS before 1957*. London: HMSO.

Webster, C. (2002) *The National Health Service – A Political History*, 2nd edn. Oxford: Oxford University Press.

Wertenbaker, L. (1980) *To Mend the Heart*. New York: Free Press.

2

Nurse prescribing – impact, education and sustainability

Pamela Campbell

Introduction

This chapter is based on my involvement with nurse prescribing – the observations I have made and the impressions I have formed. I became involved with nurse prescribing when I was first appointed as a lecturer and tasked with setting up a prescribing course for almost a thousand district nurses and health visitors in Shropshire and Staffordshire. This was a daunting prospect; however, I firmly believed that extending prescribing to nurses and health visitors would improve health care for a large number of people. My enthusiasm for the job was heightened by the fact that the government was eager to train as many non-medical prescribers as possible. The course content was largely determined by the English National Board for Nursing, Midwifery and Health Visiting, the predecessor of the Nursing and Midwifery Council (NMC). The mode of delivery, the teaching and learning methods and the personnel involved were left to the discretion of course leaders and individual organisations. Internal university approval and ENB approval was required to validate the course.

I talked to the first group of students about their expectations, what they hoped to achieve, their educational needs and how they were intending to integrate prescribing into their current roles. My vivid recollection of these nurses was their disenchantment with how few items they were able to prescribe from the Community Practitioner Formulary (CPF) and the fact that they had little choice about undertaking the prescribing role. Some students were of the opinion that much of what they were being trained to prescribe could be acquired by patients directly from chemist shops in the high streets. Many felt that the prescribing training they received was inadequate because it had no pharmacology within it; the course comprised 3 days classroom contact plus an open learning pack. While the introduction of nurse prescribing claimed to increase their professional standing, many students felt that it was, in fact, undermining their integrity and frustrating their aspirations. The echo of the disquiet that started in the classroom was soon being heard in seminars and conferences across the country. There was some discontent that district nurses and health visitors had been singled out to become prescribers when many other nurses felt they could provide considerable patient benefit if they were able to prescribe. This linked to the publication of the third Crown report, which recommended that nurse prescribing should be expanded to other nurses and indeed to other healthcare professions. It was also recognised that a far wider range of medicines should be made available, but that this would require an extended prescribing course that involved substantial pharmacology and input into clinical decision making. The Department of Health (DoH) worked closely with the NMC to produce defined outcomes and criteria for assessment.

The directives for developing extended prescribing courses were clear but still allowed for some creativity and individual interpretation across higher education institutions. This course attracted a very different type of student to the earlier (V100) prescribing course. Those who elected to become extended prescribers were experienced personnel – nurse consultants, clinical nurse specialists and advanced practitioners. Not only were they different in terms of their seniority, they were also different with respect to the expectations they held. The majority saw being able to prescribe not as an end in itself but as a means to an end. They did not see being able to prescribe as a role in itself but as one skill among many that they required to do their work. Students were keen to know how they were going to integrate prescribing into their work once they returned to practice.

While being closely involved in the nurse prescribing initiative in the West Midlands, I was also appointed Secretary of the Association of Nurse Prescribers (ANP), a position I held from 2003 to 2007. This gave me the opportunity to observe what was happening nationally and how nursing as a profession was responding to prescribing. It was apparent that the implementation of nurse prescribing was not without its problems. One of these was the assumption that because the National Health Service (NHS) operates nationwide, what was being achieved in regard to nurse prescribing in one part of the country could be achieved elsewhere. In fact, change in the NHS is dependent on many factors, including the personnel involved, the priorities that Trusts set for themselves, the career plans of individuals, and the professionals' definitions of what a good service is. I discovered that not all Trusts saw nurse prescribing as a solution to the problems they had, and even those who did were not always as forthcoming in supporting the initiative as they might have been. In the absence of organisational support and encouragement, some nurses understandably did not elect to become prescribers because they saw that other roles were more valued. My involvement with the early development of nurse prescribing led me to conclude that its success depended on four interlinked factors: the nurses themselves, the training offered, the quality of nurturing and support provided by the employing organisation, and the level of encouragement and recognition offered by nurses' immediate colleagues.

Nurse prescribing represents a major milestone in the modernisation of nursing in that it significantly extends nursing practice. It signals that access to treatment can be provided by more than one discipline, and that nurses can manage a patient's journey from problem identification to initiation (or termination) of treatment. The NHS Plan (DoH, 2000) focused on the efficient delivery of services, the choice agenda and moving care closer to patients, and this was a major driver in moving the non-medical prescribing initiative forward. In addition to contesting the medical monopoly of prescribing, the initiative has given various healthcare professionals the opportunity to develop and utilise their diagnostic and therapeutic skills.

Nurse prescribing is an innovation that has facilitated many other innovations, such as nurse-led units and clinics and nurse-led discharge; it has also further enhanced the role of nurse consultants, who are now able to initiate and manage a range of treatments. Prescribing is acknowledged as requiring an advanced set of skills; it involves assessment of presenting symptoms, clinical decision making and formulation of a working diagnosis in order to select and negotiate treatment that is right for a particular individual. This requires considerable understanding and insight into a patient's condition. It should be recognised that not all nurses will be capable of or aspire to this level of practice and responsibility. As demand for nurses continues to grow in light of our ageing population and the increased incidence of long-term conditions, the profile of nurses will broaden alongside entry criteria to the profession. This means that the number of potential nurse prescribers is likely to represent a small fraction of the overall nursing population. Nurse prescribing may therefore pave the way to a two-tier system of nursing, linking to the plans of the NMC to recognise advanced practice through a professional qualification.

The impact of prescribing within nursing

Evaluation of the pilot sites for community nurse prescribing (Luker, 1997) revealed that prescribing improved job satisfaction and was considered to enhance the status of the nursing profession. It demonstrated that suitably qualified nurses are capable of diagnostic skills previously associated only with the medical profession. The '10 key roles' for nurses outlined by the Chief Nursing Officer in the NHS Plan (DoH, 2000) included prescribing as a means by which nurses could advance services by providing more readily available care. Expanding nursing beyond its traditional boundaries is viewed as essential to facilitate the new services envisaged by the NHS modernisation agenda.

Nurse prescribing has followed a long and tortuous path after its launch in the *Community Neighbourhood Nursing Review* (DHSS, 1986). Prescribing unlocks the door to medical treatment, and it appears that some critics are doubtful whether nurses should be entering into this new territory unescorted. This nervousness is by no means limited to medical colleagues. Many doctors, in fact, support the initiative, recognising that there is a place for nurses to initiate and review treatments. Those who are not supportive tend to voice concerns about the diagnostic skills of nurses. These worries may have been justified prior to the introduction of the NMC *Standards for Prescribing* (NMC, 2006). However, the standards are clear that any nurse or midwife undertaking the prescribing course must have proven competence relating to diagnosis and assessment.

Anxiety about nurses' prescribing role remains prevalent among pharmacists and some nurse managers. Pharmacists are familiar with the medical prescribing role and are therefore unlikely to question the educational preparation for prescribing which doctors have undergone. They are also familiar with the high number of prescribing errors, near misses and adverse events linked to prescribing, and this may make them anxious about any new kind of prescriber. Some pharmacists question the length of the prescribing course for nurses (26 days of tuition plus 12 days of clinical learning). This appears very brief in comparison to their own 4 years of training in pharmacology. However, in assessing the time taken to prepare nurse prescribers, the totality of their educational and experiential learning should be considered, commencing with pre-registration training. This comprises a minimum of 7 years (3 years pre-registration training and 3 years compulsory post-registration experience) before they can apply for the prescribing course. Pharmacists frequently draw attention to the risks inherent in prescribing, and nurse managers – who are naturally risk-averse – may be influenced by their concerns and view nurse prescribing as an additional risk that has been introduced into clinical practice.

Unfortunately, there are still frequent examples of nurses who successfully gain the independent nurse prescribing qualification but do not put it into practice. The systems linked to nurse prescribing may be discouragingly unwieldy, or there may be a lack of support from managers, leading to loss of confidence. If nurses begin to question their ability to undertake independent prescribing, they may revert to asking medical colleagues to prescribe treatment that they, as nurses, would be happy to recommend. Lewin (1951) described how implementing change depends on the support of the whole organisation. Nurse prescribing has required legislation to enable it to become a reality and has therefore been driven by government policy – a top-down approach. It may be that ownership of the concept of nurse prescribing will become more widespread when the need for nurse prescribing becomes more evident at ground level – for example, as the impact of reduced hours for junior doctors (European Working Time directive) starts to be felt in 2009.

Education, roles and practice relating to nurse prescribing

Nurses make up the largest professional group within the NHS workforce. The ambitious proposals set out in the NHS plan (DoH, 2000) forced politicians to reconsider the potential of nurses and to try to unlock it through initiatives such as nurse prescribing and the creation of new roles of nurse consultants and community matrons. Policies on choice (DoH, 2003) and providing care closer to home (DoH, 2006a) accelerated the opening of the entire British National Formulary (with the exception of some controlled drugs) to independent nurse prescribers, following the introduction in 2001 of a relatively limited formulary.

Although the focus of this book, and most contemporary literature, is on independent and supplementary prescribing, it is important to remember that the vast majority of nurse prescribers are district nurses and health visitors, who were the pioneers of non-medical prescribing. These nurses are now referred to as "community practitioner" prescribers or "V100" prescribers because of their annotation on the NMC register. Independent and supplementary nurse prescribers are annotated as V300 prescribers. There are currently more than 30 000 V100 prescribers in comparison to only 8200 independent/supplementary nurse prescribers, and although the latter are growing rapidly, it will be some time before they match the number of community practitioner prescribers.

District nurse and health visitor prescribing is restricted to a limited formulary, and the underpinning education to prepare practitioners for this prescribing role was similarly limited when it was first introduced. Prescribing rates for community practitioners are much lower than anticipated, with the majority of prescribing comprising wound dressings. The reasons for low prescribing rates may be attributable to a variety of factors, including an inappropriate formulary for widespread use, lack of commitment from practitioners who were effectively conscripted into a prescribing role, lack of confidence due to limited preparation, and practical difficulties with general practices wanting to maintain control of prescribing patterns for computerised audit purposes.

Within district nursing, there has been lobbying to enable community staff nurses to prescribe. This has arisen because the specialist practice district nurses, who are community practitioner prescribers, tend to direct and oversee care, whereas the community staff nurses have more direct patient contact. This means the staff nurse is frequently the main person requiring a new supply of dressings or lotions, but she needs a nurse prescriber to prescribe these products. The NMC have agreed that community staff nurses should be eligible to become community practitioner prescribers, and appropriate training packages (which will comprise around 10 days of learning plus clinical learning) are now being determined. This new category of prescriber will have an annotation of V150 on the NMC record.

Education for nurse prescribing

Influences on prescribing education

The national rollout of community practitioner prescribing took place between 1998 and 2001, when virtually all existing district nurses and health visitors were enrolled in short educational courses which would equip them to become prescribers. This was an unprecedented move, funded centrally with £16 million of government money, to upskill a community workforce regardless of whether or not they wished to take on the additional prescribing role. The lack of any selection process was also unique; every district nurse and health visitor was deemed capable of undertaking this degree-level module regardless of how recent her previous educational study had been or at what level. All district nurses and health visitors had indeed completed some post-registration study in order to gain their HV/District Nurse qualification, but some had done this training 20 or more years earlier, when it may have been at a lower academic level. Consequently community practitioner prescribing courses were frequently attended by groups of students who were resentful and disinterested in the prescribing role. Nonetheless, fear of failure and the impact this might have on their clinical credibility appeared to spur on most of them to succeed. The ENB (which regulated nurse education at that time) deemed an unseen examination the most appropriate means of ensuring public protection in relation to these new prescribers. This encouraged cramming but did little to instil deep-seated learning.

Nurse prescribing education therefore made an ungainly entrance into the world. The need to deliver education to large numbers of post-registration community nurses/health visitors required universities to design and deliver courses quickly in order to match the service demands of the NHS. This challenged university validation processes which were charged with accommodating the demands of the Department of Health and of the nursing professional regulator, thus laying the foundation stones for future accredited education to equip NHS professionals to work in new and different ways. Education for prescribing was visualised by strategists, ratified by the professional regulator and then delivered by the universities with little leeway in how this was done. This was in contrast to the usual process, whereby universities designed courses and then sold them to the NHS.

This new way of working has caused some anxiety for universities. The latest NMC standards (NMC, 2006) continue to insist on a written examination as the means of assessment for independent and supplementary prescribing. This does not sit comfortably with many educators, who argue that examinations encourage surface rather than deep learning (Skouller, 1998). The curriculum for nurse prescribing education was developed from the top down, and nursing academics had to design modules without the benefit of having worked in a prescribing role themselves. Now that nurse prescribing is well established in different settings, it is essential to invite practising nurse prescribers to review and shape the local curriculum in the interests of educating students who are fit for practice.

The role of service providers in influencing education for prescribing

NHS Trusts need to engage with universities on a regular basis to ensure that the prescribing course is dynamic and includes appropriate content. This means taking the initiative in requesting frequent curriculum reviews to ensure confidence in local courses. Nurse lecturers frequently view prescribing courses as difficult to get right (Campbell, 2004) because of the diverse background of students who undertake the module. It is virtually impossible to teach applied therapeutics within the prescribing course unless there is a homogenous group of students with similar clinical interests. In reality, the students are likely to come from a medley of healthcare backgrounds ranging from mental health to midwifery. This makes it necessary to focus on the generic principles relating to prescribing and pharmacology, which is less satisfying for individuals who would like a course tailored to their particular needs.

Because of the generic nature of the prescribing course, nurses must employ self-directed learning or clinical learning alongside their designated medical mentor in order to increase their knowledge of the specific drugs they are likely to prescribe. This makes it vital that the suitability of mentors is assessed by employers. Learning to take the initiative in learning is appropriate because nurse prescribers will need to research new drugs and critique their effectiveness and safety as part of their on-going practice and development.

Education in context

As well as awarding academic credits, the Independent and Supplementary Nurse Prescribing Course also confers a professional qualification (recorded by the NMC), which is the licence to prescribe. It is for this reason that the prescribing course cannot comprise a larger mandatory study package that includes clinical examination, diagnostics and consultation. This is unfortunate, as the process of prescribing involves consultation, assessment, clinical decision making and finally prescribing (or recommending treatment). The NMC has attempted to address this by stipulating that nurses must have demonstrable skills in assessment prior to enrolling on a prescribing course (NMC, 2006). This means that many nurses need to access courses that equip them with assessment skills prior to applying for prescribing education, an improvement on the previous situation where nurses were *assumed* to have assessment skills when they came on the prescribing course.

The need to take an additional course focussed on assessment skills raises mentorship issues. Prescribing training requires nurses to have a designated medical practitioner of specialist registrar level or equivalent (NPC, 2005) to provide 12 days (or equivalent) of clinical tuition. In practice, this is difficult for many nurses to negotiate, particularly in the community setting. Assessment skills courses are also likely to require clinical mentorship because of the need to practice assessment in a clinical setting. The problem of finding a receptive mentor prepared to invest such a significant amount of time and effort will therefore be doubled. Combining mentorship for prescribing *and* assessment skills might be a sensible solution. However, the university modular system could struggle to cope with this amalgamation of learning. Nurse prescribing may yet again be required to test the flexibility of academic systems!

Pharmacology within nurse prescribing education

Nurses have a key role to play in the management and administration of medication, including supporting patients with long-term conditions who need to fit therapeutic regimes into their lives on an ongoing basis. This means that nurses require ownership of medicines management, yet this is still generally viewed as the prerogative of the medical profession, which points to deficits in the teaching of pharmacology to pre registration nursing students recognised both in the UK (Latter *et al.*, 2000) and internationally (Bullock & Manias, 2002). The new curriculum for pre-registration nursing will pay more attention to this in the future, making it much easier for nurses to undertake prescribing courses later in their careers. The Department of Health is ensuring that pharmacology features strongly within the nurse prescribing curriculum, possibly in response to criticism that the original programme for district nurses and health visitors contained no pharmacology.

The degree to which pharmacology is addressed in nurse prescribing courses is variable, depending on the outlook of the particular university. Such lack of parity raises concerns, particularly as the baseline knowledge of nurses embarking on a prescribing course will itself be variable, with mental health nurses, for example, likely to have less knowledge relating to co-morbidity and physiology. Unlike doctors, nurses are not required to have studied A-level (or even GCSE) chemistry, so their knowledge of molecular sciences may be limited. This worries many pharmacists who do not appreciate that nurses may be safe prescribers without having a strong scientific base. Experienced nurses taking prescribing courses have different skills from those of pharmacists or medical students. Their clinical experience means that they have observed the use of drugs in real-life situations; they are aware of the therapeutic consequences of drug treatments and the manifestations of adverse reactions; they have familiarity with drug names and drug groupings and are aware that patients cannot be categorised in relation to their medication requirements as textbooks suggest. Education about prescribing needs to be tailored to this kind of knowledge. If it takes a traditional scientific stand, it is unlikely to be well received or understood (Coleman, 2000).

The culture of nursing encourages nurses to seek advice and help from colleagues. Pharmacists can thus be reassured that nurse prescribers will be safe practitioners even though their pharmacological knowledge, in comparison to that of medical prescribers, may come from a less traditional scientific background.

Prescribing and advanced practice

Reforms across the NHS mean that nursing has been put under the spotlight to see whether it can take on roles that were traditionally in the medical domain. The introduction of nurse consultants has shown that high levels of expertise can be attained by motivated nurses equipped with vast clinical experience and a high level of theoretical knowledge gained at master's-degree level. The number of nurse consultants remains small (724 in England in 2005), but nevertheless they are, and will be essential to developing the profile of nursing. Prescribing is likely to be one of the key components of the consultant role. Although no data is available on the percentage of nurse consultants qualified as independent/supplementary prescribers, this percentage is thought to be high. Anecdotal evidence suggests that the early cohorts of nurses undertaking prescribing training contained a high proportion of nurse consultants who needed to complete the qualification promptly in order to be able to conduct their role more effectively. The steps towards becoming a consultant nurse or advanced practitioner have never been clearly defined; *Modernising Nursing Careers* (DoH, 2006b) promises to address this. It may be that a new educational infrastructure is needed to prepare the future nursing workforce and that this may be built around the three core functions identified in *Liberating the Talents* (DoH, 2002). Career pathways would be based on public health, first-contact care and long-term conditions, with prescribing education a vital component of advanced practitioner status, regardless of the clinical root.

The professional regulating body for nursing, the NMC, has been slow to define advanced practice, although this is imminent. In the absence of a clear definition, various titles and roles have emerged that lay claim to advanced practice scope or status. Any nurse working in an autonomous manner could legitimately state that she is an advanced practitioner and seek access to prescribing courses. The *Standards of Proficiency for Nurse and Midwife Prescribers* (NMC, 2006) have now clearly stated that applicants to prescribing courses must have a minimum of 3 years' post-registration experience and 'sufficient knowledge and competence to assess a patient's clinical condition'. Employers are charged with assessing this competence before supporting applications. This is reassuring, but calls into question the position of independent/supplementary nurse prescribers who qualified prior to the introduction of these standards. Employers may now consider assessing and recording the competence of existing prescribers in order to strengthen clinical governance.

The impact of prescribing on the nursing role

Nursing has always struggled to articulate its unique position in relation to medicine. Advanced nurse practitioners have been accused of trying to become 'mini doctors', and nurses have had to emphasise that care, rather than cure, and the therapeutic use of self in relation to patient care are at the heart of their role. The authority to prescribe may tempt nurses, and others, to stress the *curing* rather than the *caring* element of what they do. This blurs the boundaries between medicine and nursing. Education for nurse prescribing must raise the question, 'If doctors and nurses can both prescribe, what is the difference between them?' Many students struggle with this; yet, unless the question can be answered by each individual for herself or himself, there is a danger of the nursing ethos being subsumed within a medical role. Organisations and workforce planners should also consider this question in order to be clear about function and requirements.

It is hoped that prescribing will be viewed by nurses as a secondary rather than a primary function. They are likely to explore behaviour and lifestyle changes in preference to prescribing wherever possible. Nursing is essentially pragmatic, and this is vital in the prescribing role to improve adherence to therapeutic regimes. The relationship between nurses and their patients tends to be more equal than that between doctors and patients, with doctors traditionally adopting an authoritative stance. This means that patients may confide in nurses that they are not taking their medicines as directed (for whatever reason), when they would not tell a doctor for fear of being 'reprimanded'. The nurse prescriber, using a negotiated approach to treatment, can therefore expect to improve adherence.

Medicines management is now seen as a priority for most NHS Trusts, particularly Primary Care Trusts which are very aware of the huge financial overspend linked to non-compliance. Nurse prescribers can assist with the management of medicines in order to maximise financial resources. For example, a community nurse looking at a huge stockpile of medicines within a patient's home may realise that this has accumulated because the patient is confused between the generic name on the repeat prescription list and the trade name of the drug he or she is taking. This leads the patient to re-order all the drugs on the repeat prescription sheet, whether required or not. A simple educational intervention whereby the nurse explains the drug names to the patient, or colour codes the repeat prescription sheet and boxes of tablets, could save thousands of pounds.

New roles in healthcare

The Department of Health is promoting social enterprise as a means of bringing innovation and flexibility into healthcare, which are often inhibited by the monolithic structure of the NHS. They are seeking to support entrepreneurial nurses who can manage new services outside the NHS. Prescribing may be key in this. However, although research has demonstrated that the 'pioneering' nurse prescribers were those who had attained levels of seniority that permitted them to initiate innovative new practices (Bradley *et al.*, 2005), finding nurse-entrepreneurs among the general nursing population may be difficult. The culture of nursing discourages risk and promotes compliance, characteristics at odds with the entrepreneurial spirit! Nurse prescribers employed outside the NHS face difficulties in gaining access to NHS prescribing budgets. Although it is laudable that the government has identified nurses as a workforce capable of increasing choice within the NHS and in healthcare generally, it is important to be realistic. Despite the added value of honours degrees within nursing, nursing is not yet a graduate profession, nor it is likely to be one for the foreseeable future. The number of graduates is probably relatively small, and the majority of nurses may not be comfortable with progressing their career too far or expanding their role. Nurse prescribers are therefore likely to be exceptions to the norm, and policy based on expanding nurses' roles must be mindful of this.

National practitioner programmes are promoting a variety of non-nursing roles such as physicians' assistants (also referred to as medical care practitioners) and emergency care practitioners. These often link closely to advanced nursing practice roles. The advanced critical care practitioner (NPP/CCPB, 2006) is one example of a new career that will include prescribing but may be accessed by graduates with a non-nursing background. Although these new roles do not include prescribing authority as yet, their scope and remit suggest that this will be legislated for in the near future.

Nurse prescribing has broken the medical monopoly on prescribing, and other professional groups will follow. At present, independent prescribing for pharmacists is not fully fledged, and prescribing for allied health professionals remains at the level of supplementary prescribing requiring medical input into clinical management plans. Allied health professional prescribing is limited to physiotherapists, radiographers, podiatrists and optometrists, and there are, as yet, no signs that these practitioners are about to become independent prescribers. This presumably means that prescribing for physicians' assistants and other innovative careers is some time off. However, service demand for new roles that can be performed without medical intervention is urgent.

Operational aspects of nurse prescribing

As the number of nurse prescribers grow, the systems and infrastructure to support them will inevitably strengthen. Many nurses who undertook prescribing training soon after the introduction of independent/supplementary nurse prescribing found that they were trying to implement not only a new role but also new systems to facilitate their prescribing. This situation is improving as Trusts are beginning to acquire significant numbers of nurse prescribers who have 'tested the systems'. However, there is a continuing need to ensure that the views of nurse prescribers are represented on drug and therapeutic committees, so that prescribing at a strategic level is not dominated by doctors.

As there are far more nurses than either doctors or allied health professionals, it is reasonable to assume that the number of nurse prescribers will soon match or overtake the number of medical prescribers. This means that nurses must have equal access with doctors to continuing professional development; they must have equal influence in relation to designing systems and processes and in determining the range of drugs to be available within the Trust formulary. While this may seem reasonable, it is unlikely to happen without considerable effort owing to the strength of the medical power base that has developed over many years. Nurse prescribers are novices in the prescribing arena but need to involve themselves immediately in high-level strategic decision making if they are to make their mark. This is not an easy task for people imbued with nursing culture of 'waiting in the wings'.

Patient Group Directions

When Patient Group Directions (PGDs) were first introduced in 2002, it was not foreseen just how widely they would be adopted. Many Trusts appear to be using them almost as an alternative to nurse prescribing without perhaps fully understanding their limitations and accountability. Many nurses who use PGDs incorrectly refer to what they are doing as 'prescribing'. Administering drugs under PGDs means following a set of instructions which does not allow for creative clinical judgement and cannot meet the needs of patients who do not fit the PGD rules, as happens very frequently. Setting up PGDs is time-consuming and bureaucratic and not in tune with a health service that professes to be dynamic and influenced by patient choice. Vicarious liability is met by the employer who has a clear responsibility to train staff to use PGDs appropriately.

Pay and prescribing

Nurse prescribing has never been linked to a skills set within the *Agenda for Change* (DoH, 2004a) bandings. This thorny issue tends to be avoided by strategists working within a cash-strapped NHS, but it deserves consideration. Nursing salaries have never been comparable with medical salaries and there are good reasons for this. However, prescribing confers significantly heightened responsibility on nurses and increased risk of litigation; if nurse prescribing is linked to professional standards for advanced practice, all of these must surely strengthen the case for higher remuneration for the prescribing role. Nurse-led services that are dependent on nurse prescribing are still relatively few. However, if these were to increase, nurse prescribing could gain more widespread recognition, and both employers and the profession may find it increasingly difficult to justify no additional reimbursement.

Continuing professional development

The importance of continuing professional development (CPD) for nurse prescribers is emphasised by the NMC in order to maintain competence and enhance patient safety. The systems for CPD in relation to prescribing should already be in place for medical prescribers and it would seem unnecessary to run separate sessions for nurse prescribers, rather than holding updates for *all* prescribers. Trusts expressing concern about CPD for nurse prescribing may have realised that their current provision of on-going education for *medical* prescribers is not as robust as it should be. Prescribing is one area where multidisciplinary learning should be implemented with comparative ease. Patients receiving prescribed treatments have a right to expect that the prescriber is properly educated whether a nurse, doctor, pharmacist or allied health professional. Employers will also need to engage in on-going assessment of competence. *Agenda for Change* (DoH, 2004a) and the *Knowledge and Skills Framework* (DoH, 2004b) have strengthened the annual appraisal system for nurses, but reviewers will need to be identified who have sufficient skills to assess competence in relation to prescribing.

Nurse prescribers in the community will have their prescribing costs and the products they are prescribing tracked via PACT (prescribing analysis cost trends). These data give pharmaceutical advisors information about the amount and type of prescribing that individuals are engaged in and may give some insight into competency. Nurses prescribing in the hospital setting do not always have their prescribing tracked in the same way, and individuals may need to self-audit and discuss their prescribing with pharmacy colleagues at planned intervals. This is not entirely satisfactory as a means of ensuring competence, and organisations may seek to introduce alternative methods, such as regular reviews with pharmacists. Appropriate CPD is an important part of the risk management and quality assurance responsibilities of PCTs, practices and individual health professionals. CPD for prescribers must evolve to reflect increasing understanding of what constitutes safe practice in non-medical prescribing.

For nurses working in primary care, keeping up with new drugs is challenging, and those working with a very wide range of clients need to remain up to date across a wider spectrum of drugs than their hospital or specialist colleagues. It is unfortunate that the provision of protected learning time for prescribers does not appear to be common in NHS Trusts. Given the frequency of medication errors (National Patient Safety Agency, 2007), some of which are life-threatening, it is surprising that Trusts do not appear committed to study time that is supplementary to Post Registration Education and Practice (PREP) for nurses (NMC, 2004). This may be because extra study time means time out for prescribers and is therefore costly. However, *not* providing such study time may well prove far more costly in the long term. Prescribers' CPD could be linked to a specified pharmacist mentor who would use a case-study approach to explore the evidence base underpinning prescribing decisions. Although this would still require additional learning time, it would mean less time away from patients, and the true expertise of the pharmacist would be put to good use. Alternatively, e-learning with a designated provider could facilitate parity of standards. If all Trusts were to pool their resources for CPD for prescribing, an on-line resource could be provided, with accompanying tests for prescribers to self-assess their level of competence. For this to happen, a government or professional directive would be required.

The future non-medical prescribers

Modernising Nursing Careers (DoH, 2006b) aims to support a more structured approach to career progression within nursing. It sets a direction, places emphasis on the core values of nursing and should be used as a blueprint to link prescribing education and CPD to career progression. To date, the selection of students for prescribing courses has been based predominantly on patient need, so that nurses who could prove that they would enhance patient care by becoming prescribers were funded by Trusts or health authorities. However, central funding for non-medical prescribing is now on the wane and this may threaten the numbers of nurses, pharmacists and allied health professionals presenting as prospective prescribers. Some Trusts may now provide tuition fees, but others may feel that fees should be met by the individuals concerned as they will gain personally from holding an additional professional qualification. The danger of this is that non-medical prescribing could become dominated by career-focused nurses who see prescribing as one step on the ladder to senior positions, rather than as a means of providing a sustainable service not dependent on medical intervention. To avoid this, Trusts may decide that they need to meet education costs in full. They also need to consider succession planning and invest in sufficient non-medical prescribers to ensure continuity of service, allowing for sickness and absence, within specialty areas.

The ongoing financial crisis in the NHS means that new initiatives within nursing, such as the introduction of community matrons to manage high-intensity users of health services, frequently flounder because of lack of investment. However, the political drive behind nurse prescribing has been so unswerving that it is difficult to imagine that it too will fail to realize its potential because of lack of funding. As research and evaluation provide more evidence of its capacity to provide efficient and appropriate care, nurse prescribing should continue to flourish and expand.

Conclusion

Nurse prescribing is a key component of numerous government healthcare policies, and its scope and the extent to which it is taken up by nurses is likely to expand in the future. Its introduction has made a clear statement that medicines management falls within the nursing domain, thus blurring the boundaries between nursing and medicine. This makes it imperative that nurses be mindful of their unique contribution to care and that they do not try to become 'mini-doctors'.

It is clear that skills required for prescribing are closely related to the multiple skills required for advanced practice. It is also clear that the more complex the care patients require, the more need there is for health professionals to collaborate. Because initial preparation for prescribing may need to be differentiated according to professional discipline, Trusts should therefore adopt a collaborative approach to CPD. This would facilitate consistency, enable all prescribers to appreciate the breadth of knowledge and expertise within their organization and enhance understanding of different approaches to treatment and care.

REFERENCES

Bradley, E. J., Campbell, P. & Nolan, P. (2005) Nurse prescribers: Who are they? How do they perceive their role? *Journal of Advanced Nursing*, **51**(5), 439–48.

Bullock, S. & Manias, E. (2002) The educational preparation of undergraduate nursing students in pharmacology: a survey of lecturers' perceptions and experiences. *Journal of Advanced Nursing*, **40**(1), 7–16.

Campbell, P. (2004) Nurse prescribing: the higher education institutions' perspective. *Nurse Prescribing*, **2**(5), 194–6.

Coleman, I. (2000) Pharmacological intervention – insight into prescribing for health visiting. In: A. Robotham & D. Sheldrake (eds), *Health Visiting: Specialist and Higher Level Practice*. London: Churchill Livingstone.

Department of Health (2000) *The NHS Plan: A Plan for Investment, a Plan for Reform*. London: Department of Health.

Department of Health (2002) *Liberating the Talents: Helping Primary Care Trusts and Nurses to Deliver the NHS Plan*. London: Department of Health.

Department of Health (2003) *Building on the Best: Choice, Responsiveness and Equity within the NHS*. London, Department of Health.

Department of Health (2004a) *The NHS Knowledge and Skills Framework*. London: Department of Health.

Department of Health (2004b) *Agenda for Change; What Will It Mean for You?* London: Department of Health.

Department of Health (2006a) *Our Health, Our Care, Our Say: A New Direction for Community Services*. London: Department of Health.

Department of Health (2006b) *Modernising Nursing Careers: Setting the Direction*. London: Department of Health.

DHSS (1986) *Neighbourhood Nursing – A Focus for Care. Report of the Community Nursing Review*. Cumberlege Report. London: HMSO.

Latter, S., Rycroft-Malone, J., Yerrell, P. & Shaw, D. (2000) Evaluating educational preparation for a health education role in practice: the case of medication education. *Journal of Advanced Nursing*, **32**, 1282–90.

Lewin, K. (1951) *Field Theory in Social Sciences*. New York: Harper and Brothers.

Luker, K. (1997) *Evaluation of Nurse Prescribing. Final Report – Executive Summary.* Liverpool: University of Liverpool.

National Patient Safety Agency (2007) *Quarterly National Reporting and Learning System Data Summary.* http://www.npsa.nhs.uk/health/resources/NRLSdata (accessed 20 May 2007).

National Practitioner Programme/Critical Care Programme Board (2006) *The National Education and Competence Framework for Advanced Critical Care Practitioners.* London: Department of Health.

National Prescribing Centre (2005) *Training Non-Medical Prescribers in Practice: A Guide to Help Doctors Prepare for and Carry Out the Role of Designated Medical Practitioner.* http://www.npc.co.uk. Liverpool: National Prescribing Centre.

National Health Service (2005) Hospital and Community Health Services Non-medical Workforce Census, 30 September 2005.

Nursing and Midwifery Council (2004, revised) *The PREP Handbook.* London: NMC.

Nursing and Midwifery Council (2006) *Standards of Proficiency for Nurse and Midwife Prescribers.* London: NMC.

Skouller, K. (1998) The influence of assessment methods on students' learning approaches. *Higher Education* (Aus), **35**(4), 453–72.

3

Nurse prescribers: from 2003 to 2006

Eleanor Bradley

The conditions under which policies are conceived are often very different from those in which they are implemented. Nurse prescribing has been promoted as a way of increasing access to care for service users and of streamlining and enhancing the experience of care through the provision of a complete care package delivered by one specialist practitioner. This would appear to be an improvement on a system which necessitates making multiple appointments, having investigations carried out in different locations, seeing many different people and having no clear idea of who has overall responsibility for care. Yet an early critique of the nurse prescribing initiative (McCartney *et al.*, 1999) suggested that the drive behind nurse prescribing was not to improve the patient experience but to save money, transfer medical work to nurses and challenge the professional power of doctors. In a world where nurses spent precious time standing outside doctors' offices waiting for a prescription to be signed, the expectation was that nurses would come forward eagerly to train as prescribers.

This chapter focuses on nurses who opted to train as prescribers between 2003 and 2006. These nurses could be described as the pioneers of extended nurse prescribing, with many being the first to train in their organisations. The chapter explores whether this group shared any characteristics – such as their nursing backgrounds, personality traits or current positions – and examines their reasons for becoming prescribers, how they felt prescribing would affect their practice and how they perceived their colleagues and service users would react.

The Pioneers: who are they?

Nurse prescribing was first introduced in the UK for community nurses, who were permitted to use a very limited formulary (the Nurse Prescribing Formulary, or NPF), which enabled them to prescribe a range of dressings, ointments and creams. Luker *et al.* (1997) conducted the first evaluation of how successful this limited venture had been and it was largely on the basis of his work that nurse prescribing was eventually opened up to all nurses, working in different settings and in various specialties. Latter *et al.* (2004) conducted a national survey of 246 extended independent nurse prescribers, including an in-depth evaluation of 10 case sites. The primary purpose was to examine how nurses were utilising their extended independent prescribing roles; there was no specific focus on the role of the supplementary nurse prescriber. Indeed, most accounts of extended nurse prescribing roles have concentrated on independent rather than supplementary prescribing even though some nurses, such as those working in mental health, are totally reliant on this role in order to prescribe.

When, in 2003, supplementary prescribing was introduced for nurses working with service users diagnosed with long-term, chronic conditions, the generic independent nurse prescribing course was amended with the addition of a mere 2 days to address issues specific to supplementary prescribing. Many UK prescribing courses have remained primarily focussed on nurses intending to prescribe independently for physical conditions. Our study included *all* nurses who had opted to prescribe during a specified period of time, exploring why they had opted to prescribe, how they hoped to employ their new prescribing role and any concerns they felt or barriers they anticipated.

In 2006, nurse prescribing was extended yet further, and legislation was amended to allow nurses to prescribe from the entire British National Formulary (BNF) *within their competence and scope of practice.* Despite this revolution in the remit of the nurse prescribing role, nurse prescribing courses continue to concentrate on issues related to independent prescribing, with little time given to how supplementary prescribing could be rolled out in practice. This has become of even greater concern since allied health practitioners (AHPs) have been permitted to become supplementary prescribers.

Prescribing courses must evolve in tune with policy and practice developments in order to provide all non-medical prescribers with the knowledge and expertise they need to put prescribing into practice. Kaas (2000) stated that more information about nurse prescribers was needed to ensure that all nurses were receiving training appropriate to their level of experience and knowledge. McCann and Baker (2002) presented some preliminary data on nurses coming forward for extended independent nurse prescribing. They were between 30 and 40 years of age and had, on average, 12.8 years experience in the profession. Latter *et al.* (2004) found that the majority of nurses training as extended independent nurse prescribers were in senior positions (including nurse practitioners, specialists and managers) and predominantly worked in general practice surgeries and other primary care settings. Over half of their sample had a nursing degree and one fifth a postgraduate degree. Rafferty (1996), commenting on the nursing profession, stated that its members were predominantly female and characterised by traditional female traits such as being 'caring' and 'warm'. We wanted to investigate whether these attributes are also shared by nurses who trained in joint supplementary and extended independent nurse prescribing.

To do this, we surveyed over 400 nurses studying to become prescribers at five universities in one region of the UK.

The nurses in our sample were predominantly female (87%), with a mean age of 42 years (range 25 to 59 years). However, the early 'pioneering' cohorts of nurses, who trained between 2003 and 2004, included significantly more male nurses than might have been expected ($p = 0.03$). It is difficult to explain this as there are no data on the part gender plays in role development in nursing. It is, however, likely that males were working in areas where nurse prescribing could improve the quality of service they provided. There are also a higher proportion of male nurses working in mental health services, and this course represented the first opportunity for these nurses to qualify as supplementary prescribers. It may equally be possible that males saw this development as an opportunity to advance their careers. Organisations may also play a part in selecting people who are thought to have leadership qualities; males occupy disproportionately more senior roles in nursing than females. Similar to the findings from the study of Latter *et al.* (2004), the nurses in the sample were well educated, with 40% holding a first degree and 12% a postgraduate degree.

Criticism of nurse prescribing training has focussed on its limited duration, with only 26 days' training plus 12 days of supervised practice. Some doctors have objected that a mere 38 days of education will leave nurses unprepared for the complexities of prescribing decisions and threaten patient safety (*Pulse* newsletter, October, 2006). Nurses feel, however, that their closeness to and knowledge of patients equip them admirably for prescribing (O'Dowd, 2007). Our sample suggests that the nurses coming forward for training are very experienced, with a mean time since qualification of 18 years (range 3 to 40 years). Over 80% were senior nurses, practicing at band 7 or above, as defined by the *Agenda for Change*. They were, however, a very mobile group, having spent a mean of only 4.5 years in their current position. As data collection progressed, we noted that many nurses were coming forward to train because prescribing was a requirement of a new post or promotion. This meant that these nurses were not only implementing a new skill but also doing so on a new team. Chapter 4 ('Nurse Prescribing Observed') considers the potential impact of this situation on the successful implementation of nurse prescribing within teams.

We compared the profile of nurses who presented for prescribing training between 2003 and 2004 and those who came forward at a later stage of the nurse prescribing initiative (until late 2006). There were few differences between the nurses in terms of their educational backgrounds, experience and seniority. This finding should allay fears that opening up prescribing to larger numbers of nurses would result in less experienced nurses being accepted onto the training course. Nurses in both the early and later cohorts occupied positions of equivalent seniority, were equally experienced and had spent a similar number of years in practice. The percentage of graduate nurses in the UK has remained relatively constant over the past 15 years, with approximately 10% of nurses holding a degree (Rafferty, 1996). However, in 2005–2006, only 4% of the nurses who qualified were educated to degree level (Shields & Watson, 2007). Our sample therefore represents an extremely well-educated group of nurses, with 52% holding a first or postgraduate degree. On the face of it, these prescribers, of whom 12% held a postgraduate degree and many of whom were in senior positions, should be people capable of driving the prescribing initiative forward within their organisations.

While a principal requirement for acceptance onto the training course is the ability to study at a level equivalent to degree level, organisations should not be tempted to use this as their only selection criterion when considering applicants for prescribing training. Criteria for selecting trainees may need to include qualities as important as academic credibility or more so. For example, potential trainees must be able to demonstrate in-depth experience and knowledge of their specialty areas and be able to justify why their team will benefit from including a non-medical prescriber.

Job titles in present-day healthcare services are numerous and varied, and nurses in our study described their roles using a vast array of such titles. Many of these overlapped, so we chose to group people under the following headings: nurse specialists (28.8%); team members (28.1%); team managers (17.6%); nurse practitioners (16.2%); community nurses, including district nurse and health visitors (7.5%); and consultant nurses (1.6%). The trainee prescribers came from a range of workplace settings. Most were based either in hospital (35%) or the community (34%); a further 18% were based in general practice, and 13% described themselves as working in 'other' settings, including the prison service and private sector. We also asked nurses to state their specialty area (Table 3.1).

The nurse prescribing course clearly attracts nurses seeking to apply prescribing in very different settings. Inevitably, these nurses will have a wide range of educational needs. Although the number of nurses based in general practice was smaller overall than the number of nurses based in hospitals or the community, practice nurses represented the largest body of trainee prescribers when ranked by speciality. Some trainee prescribers were working in large multidisciplinary teams and others in relative isolation, with limited access to medical support. This has implications for the support needs of prescribers during and after training and highlights the challenges facing higher education institutions (HEIs), mentors and organisations. The issues of educational and organisational support are discussed further in Chapter 2.

Not all of the nurses in our study had expected to be studying alongside nurses from very different specialities, and many had concerns that the course was too generic to meet their needs (Bradley *et al.*, 2006). However, despite initial concerns, lecturers reported that mixed groups were ultimately perceived by students to be beneficial because they broadened discussion and helped them to consider the implementation of prescribing in a range of settings and thereby to sharpen their ideas about innovative approaches to their own prescribing practice (Bradley *et al.*, 2006).

Table 3.1 Specialty areas

Speciality	Number	Rank
General practice	83	1
Mental health	52	2
District nursing	32	3
General hospital/acute care	24	4
Diabetes	22	5
Cardiology	17	6
Community nursing	17	6
Intermediate care	12	7
Learning disability	12	7
Palliative care	11	8
Paediatrics	11	8
Neonatal	11	8
Advanced nursing practice	9	9
Older age nursing	9	9
Oncology	9	9
Sexual health	8	10
Gynaecology	8	10
A&E	7	11
Neurology	7	11
Nurse-led clinics	7	11
Orthopaedics	7	11
Respiratory	6	12
Rheumatology	6	12
Pain	4	13
Anti-coagulant therapy	4	13
Gastroenterology	4	13
Haematology	4	13
Health visiting	4	13
Public health nursing	4	13
Prison nursing	3	14
Renal	3	14
Chronic disease	2	15
Dermatology	2	15
Parkinson's disease	2	15
School nursing	2	15
Substance misuse	2	15
Occupational health	1	16
Colorectal	1	16
Ear, nose & throat	1	16
Epilepsy	1	16
Midwifery	1	16
Urology	1	16

Many nurses opt to prescribe so that they can offer patients a complete package of care and facilitate speedy access to treatment. However, the success of prescribing in these respects is dependent to a large extent on the location of the service and/or nursing professional. Service users prefer to receive care at their local general practitioner (GP) practice or in their own home because this means less time spent travelling, reduced costs and the reassurance of a familiar setting (for further discussion, see Chapter 5). If the nurse prescriber is located outside the service user's community in a hospital, access to treatment will not be improved; yet only 18% of trainee prescribers in our study were based in a GP practice. The high number of nurses based in hospital settings (35%) does not reflect the original intentions of policy makers (i.e. that nurses would be prescribing independently in general practice or as supplementary prescribers, working in the community with service users diagnosed with long-term, complex conditions). Implementing nurse prescribing in hospitals has been challenging, and some nurses have struggled to find an appropriate niche for their new skills (see Chapter 4 for more detail about the experiences of prescribers in practice).

The supplementary prescribing role has been designed specifically for nurses working with service users diagnosed with chronic conditions and is unsuitable for a triage or one-stop service. Nurses working in the community could use supplementary alongside independent prescribing, depending on their areas of specialty, to realise a flexible way of caring for their service users. In the field of mental health, supplementary prescribing is the only way in which nurses can currently work as prescribers (although with recent changes to legislation, and future extensions to the nurse prescribing role, this is likely to change). Mental health nurses across the UK have been relatively slow to take up prescribing. However, in our sample, mental health nursing was the second highest ranking nursing specialty, including 52 nurses. This was largely due to one particularly supportive mental healthcare Trust in the region where our study was based. The nurses were all based in the community, in teams that did not necessarily have access to full-time medical support or include other non-medical prescribers. As such, these trainees were facing the likelihood of working in isolation and of possibly encountering demands from service users to prescribe for conditions co-existing with their mental health condition. Nurses who will be working in such situations need help to plan how they will utilise prescribing in their practice and how they will get support in their different prescribing roles both from mentors and peers.

Often, national policies and targets look very different when applied in the local context, and nurse prescribers may not be the people whom it was anticipated would come forward for prescribing. Educational courses for healthcare workers are designed on the basis of government policy. In the case of non-medical prescribing, a much wider range of nurses has presented for training than was expected, and the course has had to expand and develop in order to meet the needs of nurse who are not working autonomously in general practice,

Table 3.2 Key skills

Key skills	Number	Rank
Interpersonal skills (communication, listening, negotiation)	348	1
Specialist knowledge (including evidence-based practice and clinical skills)	120	2
Assessment and diagnosis	97	3
Organisational skills (including time and caseload management)	64	4
Educational	41	5
Decision making	20	6
Leadership and managerial skills	16	7
Team working	11	8
Advocacy and liaison (with professionals and patients)	10	9
Risk management	8	10
Medication management	7	11
Autonomous working	6	12
Care co-ordination	5	13
Health promotion	4	14
Holistic care	3	15
Evaluation	1	16

running nurse-led clinics, or managing service users diagnosed with long-term chronic conditions. Educators will need to reflect on the needs of each new cohort of trainee prescribers and tailor their courses on each occasion to ensure that nurses feel appropriately informed and skilled for prescribing in their unique circumstances of practice.

Skills base of trainee prescribers

An oft-quoted concern about nurse prescribing is that it will move nurses away from their key role of 'caring' for patients and bring them closer to the medical role of 'curing' (Hilton, 1997; Baumann *et al.*, 1998; McCann & Baker, 2002). By taking on prescribing, nurses are accused of 'medicalising' the nursing profession, focussing increasingly on episodic, medical tasks rather than on continuous caring activities (Baumann *et al.*, 1998). In order to explore whether qualifying as a prescriber might bring about a fundamental reorientation in nursing, we asked trainee prescribers to outline the two skills that they felt underpinned their current nursing roles (Table 3.2).

Participants in our study still considered traditional 'caring' skills as the essential underpinning of their current roles, including interpersonal skills such as communication, listening and negotiation. This would suggest that nurses continue to align themselves with what might be described as their 'historical' role as carers. And it is vital that nurses retain these skills once they start prescribing. Good communication is essential to achieve concordance with treatment regimens. Many service users complain that they don't feel doctors spend enough time talking to them about their treatment options, symptoms or medication. Nurses' understanding of the importance of communication suggests that they are well placed to talk to service users about prescribing decisions. One of the proposed benefits of nurse prescribing for service users with chronic conditions is that all of their care will be provided by one person. Nurses should, therefore, be able to integrate their 'caring' and 'curing' skills and promote holistic treatment for service users, taking their feelings about medicines and treatment into consideration when making prescribing decisions, and improving their satisfaction with care and treatment. Nurses' 'caring' approach to 'curing' may be what is needed to improve concordance. Whereas doctors' involvement in care is often by necessity episodic, nurses must make sure that they value and retain their continuity of care.

Naturally, the fact that nurses in our study ranked interpersonal skills highly in their current role does not mean that every one possessed good communication skills. The importance of communicating with service users about their treatment and prescribing decisions still needs to be highlighted during prescribing training to ensure that all nurses realise the centrality of listening to service users' concerns about their treatment and symptoms and can factor these into decisions about treatment. Furthermore, emphasis should be placed on the role of nurses as health promoters and talking to service users about means of preventing future disease through maintenance of 'healthy' activities. Our findings suggest that nurses do not currently prioritise their role in promoting health (ranked as number 14).

Only one nurse stated that evaluation skills were important in her current role. While nursing is developing new roles, evaluation of their impact in practice is important if organisations are to be fully informed in deciding whether to send nurses on advanced-level courses and considering how to place nurse education and development within strategic organisational planning. Nurses are fully able to evaluate the impact of prescribing on their practice but will only do so if they appreciate the importance of critical appraisal in enhancing their practice. It is not necessary, nor is there time, to include a programme on audit and research within the nurse prescribing course; however, all prescribers should be equipped with critical appraisal skills to evaluate the impact of innovative practices.

In our study, nurses felt that they lacked knowledge of research methods and critical appraisal. Seventy per cent felt that they would require support in conducting research, and 75% felt they needed help when critically appraising studies in nursing and medical journals, which often employ complex research designs. It may not be the responsibility of higher education institutions to provide nurses with these skills; local research and development (R&D)

Table 3.3 Current involvement with medication and prescribing

Rank	Comment	Number
1	Provide expert advice (to GPs, SHOs, patients)	261
2	Act as a patient advocate: eliciting patient preferences, discussion and negotiation re: care and prescribing decisions; first point of contact for patient; utilise relationship with patient to inform prescribing decisions	128
3	Prescribing 'by proxy'/titration of doses	54
4	Assessment	39
5	Medication management (including concordance, monitoring impact, review)	38
6	Already prescribing from NPF or PGDs	36
7	Running nurse-led clinics and initiatives	20
8	Diagnosis	14
9	Providing information about alternative medication and treatment options	6

departments should be supporting all advanced-level nurses in their organisations to become research-aware. Peer support sessions are a forum for communicating the results of evaluation conducted in practice areas, and also for discussing new practices and interventions within specialty areas.

We asked nurses to describe how involved they were currently with medication and prescribing (Table 3.3).

Participants felt they already had considerable experience and expertise with respect to medicines, and it is likely that their interest in and involvement with medication were key factors in their application for prescribing training. Thirty-one per cent of our participants felt they had an important role to play in discussing medicines with service users, particularly in advocacy-type roles. Our findings suggest that for many nurses, the prescribing qualification formally acknowledges a role that they have already put into practice within their teams. Nurses may elect to become prescribers because they want this acknowledgement and the legal protection that accompanies it. Nurses assume responsibility for all information that they provide to service users about medication, even if they are recommending medication that can be bought over the counter (OTC). In the event of adverse reactions, the nurse providing the advice could be held responsible. Therefore, writing prescriptions formally may be safer for nurses because they can document their decisions and the explanations they give to service users and enjoy indemnity cover in the event of legal action. To advance their status, nurses need a formal qualification rather than continuing, as they have done historically, to discuss medication with patients, make recommendations and issue requests that their recommendations be authorised by a doctor's signature on a prescription.

In the United Kingdom, the Department of Health is currently encouraging healthcare professionals to be entrepreneurs in terms of providing care in innovative ways and initiating new practices and roles. Nurses represent the largest workforce in the National Health Service (NHS) and are therefore the key to the success of this agenda. In some of the states in the United States, nurse practitioners provide autonomous, independent services to users and design the services they offer to suit their clientele. The potential for nurses in the UK to revolutionise the way they work is huge. Prescribing represents an opportunity for nurses to seize clinical autonomy and provide a complete range of services to users. This will be particularly welcome in teams and specialities where the medical workforce is limited, where there are difficulties in providing out-of-hours care for service users and where there are service users with certain social problems, such as being homeless or a refugee.

The fear that nurse prescribers will prioritise 'curing' above 'caring' is fuelled by the assumption that prescribing will become a large part of nurses' future role, and that they will have less time to spend talking to service users about their health and treatment. However, findings from our trainee nurse prescribers suggested that they were already heavily involved in medication-related care. Half felt that they spent time on medication several times a day, and a further 35% that they were spending time, at least on a daily basis, on medication-related care. Interestingly, nurse trainees coming forward as 'pioneers' between 2003 and 2004 differed from the later cohort (2005–2006) in that they felt they spent significantly more time on both medication-related care and contributing to prescribing decisions than the earlier cohort. It would appear that as prescribing is rolled out across organisations, more nurses who frequently spend time prescribing 'by proxy' have come forward for training. Our findings would support the literature that has suggested that nurses coming forward for prescribing training are already 'experts' in medication-related issues and already contributing to prescribing decisions, albeit 'informally'. Therefore, taking on prescribing as a qualified practitioner will not be an entirely new role for nurses. Provided that they continue to prioritise their interpersonal skills whilst implementing skills more traditionally associated with a medical model of care, it should be possible for them to integrate 'caring' and 'curing' and provide service users with a holistic package of care. It remains to be seen whether nurses can maintain this balance once they incur the additional workload associated with prescribing and whether they will initiate new services to improve users' access to medicines (e.g. nurse-led clinics and triage). If nurses lose the time they have traditionally spent with service users discussing their concerns, it is difficult to see how nurse prescribing would differ from medical prescribing.

In the UK, nurses need to be nominated for the prescribing course by their employers. Some asked to be considered for the course, but a survey of independent nurse prescribers carried out in 2004 found that managers had selected the majority for training (Latter et al., 2004). In 2002, government announced that it hoped to reach a target of 10 000 nurses prescribing as independent and supplementary prescribers by 2004, raising fears that, as had happened with early community nurse prescribing, some nurses would be told to do the course in order that their organisations could be seen to be engaging with this initiative (O'Dowd, 2001) rather than being selected for their potential to streamline care and improve service users' satisfaction. Gibson *et al.* (2003) suggested three criteria for prioritising nurse prescribing trainees:

- Nurses running their own clinics or services
- Nurses working in isolation from other prescribers
- Nurses who could complete episodes of care by prescribing. (Gibson *et al.*, 2003)

University criteria focus primarily on the student's ability to study at level 3 (degree level). We asked participants in our study who had initiated their application to train as prescribers and found that over half (51%) had requested to be put forward; just under a third (32%) had been put forward by their managers, and 13% had been put forward by another colleague. It is important that all applicants for prescribing training are clear about how prescribing could help them develop their practice – that they are currently occupying roles to which prescribing is relevant and that they are working in teams which are supportive of prescribing, particularly if they are hoping to implement a supplementary prescribing role. The availability of supportive and accessible mentors is also important, and this should be given careful consideration when nurses apply for prescribing training.

Interviews with nurse lecturers teaching on prescribing courses (Bradley *et al.*, 2006) found that they felt the selection process was ad hoc and that this had serious consequences for the students. Some students were considered to struggle with the academic requirements of the course, despite having given evidence of previous study equivalent to level 3. Difficulties with the academic content of the course were described as a primary reason for nurses dropping out. Others found university approaches to learning, such as reflective writing and portfolio work, too challenging. Senior nurses sometimes had problems with the course because many had not studied in a university setting for a long time and some had completed all their previous training in practice. There was the additional exacerbation of studying alongside more junior staff and a consequent desire not to lose face. Lecturers have an important role to play in developing selection criteria and perhaps in identifying suitable students for prescribing training. Bradley *et al.* (2006) suggest that lecturers could be involved in interviewing applicants to help identify potential problem areas and signpost them, when appropriate, to introductory information and study skills materials.

Expectations of future prescribing roles

As well as looking at the characteristics of nurse prescribing trainees, we were interested in finding out how they anticipated their new prescribing role would

Table 3.4 Why did you become interested in nurse prescribing?

Comment	Number	Rank
To improve patient care generally (speeding up care, giving patients choice)	124	1
Professional and role development	73	2
To achieve autonomous practice	63	3
Mandated to attend the course/course completion was a requirement of new post	45	4
To be able to 'complete' care and improve continuity	43	5
To formalise and extend current prescribing practice (including prescribing 'by proxy')	41	6
Skills and knowledge development	34	7
To develop services (including nurse-led services)	31	8
To advance practice	22	9
To provide holistic care	19	10
To improve time management	12	11
Lack of doctors available to prescribe	8	12
Felt frustrated that couldn't prescribe	7	13

be put into practice; whether they felt that prescribing was likely to change the nature of their work; and how they felt that being a prescriber would impact on team members, service users and themselves personally. One of the reasons that nurse prescribing has been promoted is that nurses have 'close and continuing' contact with service users, placing them in an excellent position to make accurate assessments of their needs (Luker *et al.*, 1998). They 'know' their service users and can give due consideration to the social context of their lives (Russell *et al.*, 2003). District nurses have reported that being able to take responsibility for the whole process of diagnosis, prescribing and follow-up has contributed to the development of their competence and sense of professionalism (Wilhelmsson & Foldevi, 2003).

Yet nurses should not be treated as a homogenous group when considering their needs and expectations. They have different motives for their choice of profession, and their motivation to develop their practice will be related to the external and internal rewards of their work – such as intellectual stimulation and feeling useful and appreciated (Stark *et al.*, 2002). Table 3.4 outlines why nurses in our study developed an interest in prescribing.

Nurses' principal reason for becoming interested in prescribing was the improvement of patient care, in particular, access to care and patient choice. Prescribing was seen as a means of developing clinical autonomy and the ability to complete episodes of care without the necessity for medical input. Participants felt that for service users being discharged from hospital into the community, the ongoing attention of a nurse able to work across these two settings would be particularly valuable.

Personal and professional development was an often-cited reason for undertaking prescribing (see also Bradley *et al.*, 2005). As a group of nurses engaging with an initiative at an early stage of its development, it might be expected that at least a proportion would be 'high flyers', keen to develop their roles in new ways and advance professionally. Our findings would suggest that this is indeed the case. This could be a positive finding for non-medical prescribing because these nurses will be keen to advance their roles in the future. However, the desire to develop professionally could also explain the mobility of these participants. Non-medical prescribing will be difficult to sustain if nurses who complete the course leave their teams and services to gain promotion shortly after qualifying. This is particularly problematic if senior nurses are promoted to managerial roles on the basis of their prescribing qualification and subsequently have little or no clinical contact. The removal of senior nurse prescribers from teams will impoverish the guidance available to other team members interested in becoming prescribers and reduce the support available for the team's existing non-medical prescribers. Such a situation highlights the difficulties for organisations in selecting nurses for prescribing training; although it is important that candidates have the experience to take the course, it is also important to consider whether they are likely to be promoted out of their prescribing role post-qualification.

An important finding from our study of this pioneering group of nurses is that many undertook the prescribing course because it was a requirement of a new post or of another qualification that they were taking (e.g. an MSc course). Many nurses who opt to prescribe also follow other paths in further education to increase their skills and be able to expand their nursing role. For advanced practitioner courses, there is a clear need for nurses to be able to prescribe because they will be developing new services, practising autonomously and taking responsibility for auditing the impact of nurse-led care. Some nurses may be sent on the course because they have joined a team that requires all nurse team members to be prescribers or so that they can become the only nurse prescriber in the team. The success of nurse prescribing will depend on more rigorous workforce planning, addressing specific questions such as:

- Which teams will benefit from having nurse prescribers?
- What is the appropriate number of prescribers within a team?
- How can nurse prescribers be supported within teams?
- How could a nurse prescriber working in isolation be supported?

Perceived impact of prescribing

As part of looking at their expectations of prescribing, we asked trainees to consider how being able to prescribe would affect them personally (Table 3.5).

Table 3.5 How will becoming a prescriber alter your self-perception?

	Number	Rank
Increase confidence as a practitioner	74	1
Increase accountability and responsibility	48	2
Increase knowledge and skills	35	3
Increase autonomy	35	4
Become more critical of prescribing decision making (and maybe more cautious and safe)	24	5
Feel that skills and knowledge have been recognised	21	6
Feel able to improve care delivery and develop practice	20	7
Increase self-awareness and reflective practice	14	8
Enhance status	12	9
Increase job satisfaction	7	10
Increase awareness of legal issues and prescribing	6	11
Develop role	6	11
Able to consolidate and extend existing roles	3	12
Proud of attainment	3	12
Feel a more competent practitioner	3	12

Nurses anticipated that prescribing would increase their confidence as practitioners and enhance their status. They recognised that prescribing would require them to become more accountable and responsible for their practice but would also enable them to practice more autonomously.

Trainees from 2005 to 2006 were more likely than those from 2003 to 2004 to believe that their colleagues would view them differently as a result of their becoming prescribers. Early trainees were likely to be the first in their organisations and teams to undertake prescribing training. As such, they had no clear picture of the impact that prescribing might have on them and their colleagues. By contrast, many of the trainees who opted to prescribe later in the initiative had witnessed the rolling out of non-medical prescribing within their organisations and teams. Watching non-medical prescribing colleagues adapt to their new roles and assume responsibility and autonomy for their prescribing practice would have provided material for reflection on the changes that prescribing brings in terms of self-perception and the way in which prescribers are perceived by colleagues. Table 3.6 describes how trainees from the later cohort felt they would be perceived by their colleagues post-qualification.

In general, trainee prescribers felt that team members would regard their new role positively. They felt that they were already respected across the teams for their knowledge of medicines and that their potential for developing services would now be recognised. However, they were concerned that colleagues might have exaggerated expectations of their prescribing role and that there was the potential for the role to be abused. There were some fears that non-prescribing nursing colleagues might feel threatened, particularly if they occupied positions

Table 3.6 How do you expect colleagues will view you once you become a nurse prescriber?

Comments	Number	Rank
I will be utilised more widely as a resource (particularly for information and advice re medicines)	47	1
My increased knowledge and responsibility will be acknowledged (enhanced status)	37	2
Team members may have unrealistic expectations of the new role	31	3
I will be seen as altering and enhancing practice across teams, particularly through ability to 'complete' care episodes	19	4
I will be asked to write prescriptions	18	5
I may be utilised in preference to a doctor	14	6
Colleagues may feel threatened by the new role	10	7
My workload will increase as I will be utilised more widely by team	8	8
I will be asked by colleagues to take a more active role in the care of service users across the teams	6	9
I may be pressured by colleagues to act outside my scope of practice	6	9
Doctors will expect more from me	5	10
I will be seen as a role model by nursing colleagues	4	11
I will be the only nurse prescriber in the team so will be occupying a little understood role	3	12

senior to that of the prescriber. Some of the participants in our study described how non-prescribing nurse colleagues had expressed concerns that introducing a prescribing nurse into the team would lead to all nurses being required to train as prescribers, regardless of their desire to do so.

The majority of trainee prescribers (62%) felt that they would be perceived differently by service users once qualified. In particular, the nurses felt that service users would recognise their ability to prescribe as a means of gaining faster access to medicines. Some were concerned that service users might ask them to prescribe outside of their sphere of competence and request medication that their doctor had refused to prescribe. Some trainees (n = 11) were concerned that the introduction of non-medical prescribing would confuse service users who would not be able to distinguish between prescribing nurses, non-prescribing nurses and doctors. Nonetheless, despite these concerns, trainees were of the opinion that their new role would be highly regarded by service users and that they would gain credibility with them and be recognised as autonomous practitioners. They felt that service users would recognise the introduction of nurse prescribing as an attempt to improve care and services. Interestingly, nearly 40% of trainees felt that becoming a qualified prescriber would not affect the way that service users perceived them. This may be because service users were used to seeing them providing advice about medicines and prescribing 'by proxy'.

Table 3.7 Concerns about nurse prescribing

Comments	Number	Rank
Being supported in practice (including there being appropriate policies in place)	71	1
Responsibility and accountability (fear of making a mistake)	48	2
Being sufficiently knowledgeable	35	3
Time/workload issues	33	4
Legal issues, litigation and safety	32	5
How to implement prescribing	32	5
Misconceptions of role by team members (exaggerated expectations, potential for abuse of role)	28	6
Access to CPD/keeping up to date	25	7
The limited formulary	24	8
Acceptance by medical colleagues	23	9
The CMP	19	10
Lack of remuneration (and lack of recognition within AFC)	17	11
Identifying and working within scope of practice (and resisting pressure from others to prescribe outside of it)	12	12
Feeling confident enough to prescribe	10	13
Concerns as to whether the nursing role would be lost	7	14
Being a 'pioneer' (working in isolation)	5	15
Extending and changing current role	4	16
Concerns about the motivation for introducing nurse prescribing (driven by politics, doctor shortages)	3	17

Concerns about prescribing

Eighty per cent of the participants had concerns about their future prescribing role (n = 342) (Table 3.7).

These participants included some of the very first nurses in the UK to complete the course in 2003, so it is not surprising that they had some concerns about their new role. They were most worried about the commitment of their organisations to supporting them post-qualification. They wanted reassurance in particular that organisations would put policies in place to support non-medical prescribing practice. Trainees were also concerned as to whether they had sufficient knowledge to be able to prescribe. (However, it should be borne in mind that our survey was carried out at an early stage of the training course when participants might be expected to feel uncertain about their knowledge base.) They were clearly in need of some reassurance, especially given that the aim of the training course is not to provide nurses with a complete understanding of prescribing in their individual specialities but rather to convey generic prescribing principles to be applied by nurses within their own areas. This is an additional reason for organisations being seen to be committed to supporting nurses with ongoing education and development around prescribing so that prescribers can feel reassured that they will be supported during the early stages of their practice.

Trainees felt concerned about the responsibility they were taking on as prescribers and were very mindful of issues around prescribing safety and litigation. Their cautious attitude will hopefully encourage them to scrutinise prescribing decisions carefully, including instances when the appropriate decision is not to prescribe. Naturally the participants in our study were anxious about integrating their new role into their daily workload and into existing systems, particularly because they were not going to have any extra time (or indeed remuneration) to do so. Organisations might show their appreciation for the nurses taking on the role of prescriber by offering them protected time for continuing professional development (CPD) and organising seminars and presentations given by, and bringing together, non-medical prescribing colleagues. As well as demonstrating the organisation's commitment to non-medical prescribing, this would allow nurses the opportunity to offer feedback on their experiences of implementing prescribing, highlight training needs, identify how to overcome barriers within the workplace and consider how prescribers could be supported in their new roles.

Preparation

We asked the nurses participating in our study to outline what kind of training they felt would be particularly important for their prescribing practice (Table 3.8).

The nurses were clearly acutely aware of the responsibility of being prescribers and wanted knowledge of how to practice safely and within the law. They were concerned about their knowledge of pharmacology (including pharmacodynamics and pharmacokinetics) and their ability to perform drug calculations accurately. When we later asked the nurses whether they felt they would need CPD support in the area of pharmacology, 95% responded that they would. Concern about knowledge of pharmacology links with concerns about assessment skills, diagnosis and physiology. Over the last two decades, nurse training has increasingly promoted and taught a psychosocial approach to care, with less emphasis on biology, physiology and pharmacology and more on communication and interpersonal skills (Courtenay, 2002). Some educators have argued that this focus on the social and behavioural sciences has been too much at the expense of biology (Brooks et al., 2001). This shift has important implications if nurses are now being encouraged to expand their roles beyond those traditionally associated with nursing and into areas traditionally associated with medicine. The integration of key nursing skills, such as communication, with the more technical skills of prescribing is essential before a more holistic approach to patient care can become a reality.

Table 3.8 Most important training needs

Training needs	Number	Rank
Pharmacology (including pharmacodynamics, kinetics, drug actions)	264	1
Legal issues	151	2
Assessment	70	3
Clinical and practical applications of prescribing	58	4
Role boundaries and scope of practice	45	5
Ethics of prescribing	45	5
The Clinical Management Plan	35	6
Anatomy and physiology	31	7
Accountability	23	8
Future support for prescribing	21	9
Diagnosis	16	10
Safety and prescribing	15	11
Politics and policy issues	6	12
Drug calculations	5	13
Reflective practice	5	13
Patient Group Directives	5	13
Medicines management	4	14
Implementation in specific areas	4	14
Chronic disease management	3	15
Competency issues	2	16
Communication	1	17
Chemistry	1	17
Time management	1	17
Service user expectations	1	17
Cost of prescribing and drug budgets	1	17
Audit	1	17
Health psychology	1	17

According to Leathard (2001), there are three aspects of practice pertaining to pharmacology:

1. A health education role in providing advice and information to patients about their treatments
2. A responsibility to administer appropriate medicines correctly
3. The identification and evaluation of adverse drug effects at the earliest possible opportunity

Prescribing includes taking responsibility for assessment and diagnosis, and the nurses in our study were fully aware of this. Although in supplementary prescribing, that responsibility is shared with a medical prescriber, independent nurse prescribers need to be confident that they have completed a thorough assessment with the service user and made an accurate diagnosis before prescribing. Until recently in the UK, the prescribing course required trainees to be selected on the basis that they *already* possessed good assessment skills. However, the Nursing and Midwifery Councils (NMC) standards and competencies for the prescribing course place great emphasis on nurses demonstrating assessment and numeracy skills. Many prescribing courses are therefore now offering modules on assessment, which trainees must complete before or after their training. As part of prescribing examinations, nurses are being tested on their ability to carry out drug calculations and must score 100% in order to qualify.

While some of the training issues highlighted by the nurses in our study have now been addressed nationally, the medical profession continues to be concerned as to whether prescribing training for nurses is adequate (*Pulse*, 2006). It would appear that nurses share some of these concerns, and there have been calls from the nursing profession to re-examine the selection process for nurse prescribers and/or to include further training on pharmacology and other key medical skills in nursing pre-registration courses. This would require an extension of the current pre-registration programme and a refocusing of the curriculum (Scott, 2002). In Australia and Canada, nurse practitioners take on the responsibility for diagnosis and treatment, including prescribing, but they are educated to master's degree level and supported by intensive in-service education and outreach programmes (Shields & Watson, 2007). Although prescribing courses in the UK do expect nurses to be experienced, there is no uniform approach adopted by organisations or universities to identifying the abilities and knowledge of nurses applying for training. Trainees are not explicitly tested on their assessment or diagnostic skills before qualifying. It remains to be seen whether this has consequences for the safety of nurse prescribing, for the confidence of prescribers and for how many nurses put their prescribing qualification into practice.

Mentors/clinical tutors

The mentoring/clinical tutor role is fundamental to the nurse prescribing initiative. Trainees are required to have a mentor who will supervise their 12 days of training practice and formally assess their knowledge and skills. Mentors are currently medical prescribers and are advised (but not required) to attend a brief university-based training course to prepare them. Some mentors are more experienced in working with nurses than others; as more nurses take prescribing training, they are more likely to have a mentor who has previously supervised nurse prescribers. It is recommended that in order to meet the contact time requirement, mentors should be based locally, and many nurses select mentors with whom they already have a good working relationship. Mentors are primarily responsible for providing nurses with prescribing training specific to their specialty area and for helping them consider how they will apply prescribing principles in practice. In our study, the majority of nurses (82%) who trained

Table 3.9 How did you select your mentor?

Selection criteria	Number	Rank
Good working relationship	167	1
Clinical contact in workplace	54	2
Allocated to me	48	3
Already acted as mentor for previous/ongoing courses	28	4
Knowledge and experience	24	5
Recommended by a colleague	21	6
Volunteered for the role	18	7
Approachable	13	8
Only mentor available	11	9
Willing and available	9	10
Highly respected	9	10
Interested in and knowledgeable about nurse prescribing	8	11

between 2003 and 2004 got their first choice of mentor, but this was less true of the 2005–2006 cohort. Being allocated their first choice of mentor depended on how many nurses in their team were training as prescribers, how many nurses' mentors were willing to take on, how many mentors were available locally and how much support was available to them from the local university. We asked the nurses to describe how they selected their mentors (Table 3.9).

Mentors were selected mainly on the basis of accessibility and availability. Nurses preferred to be working alongside their mentors, as this enabled them to maximise the experience they could gain from clinical contact. They were also inclined to select mentors with whom they, or a colleague, had already established a good working or mentoring relationship. This was perhaps more important than the mentor's knowledge or interest in nurse prescribing.

Nurses want a high level of contact from their mentors during training. Fifteen per cent of the nurses in our study wanted to see their mentors daily, 12% wanted contact three to four times a week and the rest wanted contact at least once a week. This means that nurses need to be based close to their mentors so that travel time is reduced to a minimum. It also means that mentors need to think carefully about how many trainees they can take on, particularly as the demand for mentoring increases.

Some nurses felt that they had no choice in their mentor, and the ad hoc way in which much mentoring is organised has been criticised (O'Dowd, 2007). Nurses do need to have a good relationship with their mentors and feel able to engage in discussion about a wide range of prescribing issues. If the relationship between nurse and mentor does not allow for this, nurses may struggle to develop the confidence to apply their prescribing qualification in practice. It is not required that nurses continue their relationship with their mentor post-qualification; however, if it does continue, it could be invaluable in terms of offering support and enhancing awareness of and interest in non-medical prescribing across teams. Discussion about prescribing across teams has been found to help nurse prescribers manage feelings of uncertainty (Luker *et al.*, 1998). Otway (2001) found that many nurse prescribers believed that clinical supervision would help them to improve their prescribing practice but were not able to access it because of staffing shortages. Allowing nurses to select their mentors on the basis of good working relationships and accessibility will make it more likely that the mentoring relationship continues post-qualification.

REFERENCES

Baumann, A. O., Deber, R. B., Silverman, B. E. & Mallette, C. M. (1998) Who cares? Who cures? The ongoing debate in the provision of healthcare. *Journal of Advanced Nursing*, **28**(5), 1040–5.

Bradley, E. J., Blackshaw, C. & Nolan, P. (2006) Nurse lecturers' observations on aspects of nurse prescribing training. *Nurse Education Today*, **26**, 538–44.

Bradley, E. J., Campbell, P. & Nolan, P. (2005) Nurse prescribers: Who are they? How do they perceive their role? *Journal of Advanced Nursing*, **51**(5), 439–48.

Brooks, N., Otway, C., Rashid, C., Kilty, E. & Maggs, C. (2001) The patient's view: the benefits and limitations of nurse prescribing. *British Journal of Community Nursing*, **6**(7), 342–8.

Courtenay, M. (2002) Nurse prescribing: implications for the life sciences in nursing curricula. *Nurse Education Today*, **22**, 502–6.

Gibson, F., Khair, K. & Pike, S. (2003) Nurse prescribing: children's nurses' views. *Pediatric Nursing*, **15**(1), 20–4.

Hilton, P. (1997) Theoretical perspectives of nursing: a review of the literature. *Journal of Advanced Nursing*, **26**, 1211–20.

Kaas, M. J., Dehn, D., Dahl, D., Frank, K., Markley, J. & Hebert, P. (2000) A view of prescriptive practice collaboration: Perspectives of psychiatric-mental health clinical nurse specialists and psychiatrists. *Archives of Psychiatric Nursing*, **14**(5), 222–34.

Latter, S., Maben, J., Myall, M., Courtenay, M., Young, A. & Dunn, N. (2004) *An Evaluation of Extended Formulary Independent Nurse Prescribing: Final Report*. University of Southampton and Department of Health.

Leathard, H. (2001) Understanding medicines: conceptual analysis of nurses' needs for knowledge and understanding of pharmacology (part 1). *Nurse Education Today*, **21**, 266–71.

Luker, K. (1997) *Evaluation of Nurse Prescribing. Final Report*. Liverpool: University of Liverpool and University of York.

Luker, K. A., Austin, L., Hogg, C., Ferguson, B. & Smith, K. (1998) Nurse–patient relationships: the context of nurse prescribing. *Journal of Advanced Nursing*, **28**(2), 235–42.

McCann, T. V. & Baker, H. (2002) Community mental health nurses and authority to prescribe medications: the way forward? *Journal of Psychiatric and Mental Health Nursing*, **9**, 175–82.

McCartney, W., Tyrer, S., Brazier, M. & Prayle, D. (1999) Nurse prescribing: radicalism or tokenism? *Journal of Advanced Nursing*, **29**(2), 348–54.

O'Dowd, A. (2001) Frustration at limit of reform. *Nursing Times*, **97**, 4.

O'Dowd, A. (2007) The power to prescribe. *Nursing Times*, **103**(3), 16–18.

Otway C. (2001) Informal peer support: a key to success for nurse prescribers. *British Journal of Community Nursing*, **6**(11), 586–91.

Pulse newsletter (2006) Survey: nurse prescribing a threat to patient safety. *Pulse*, 5 October.

Rafferty, A. M. (1996) *The Politics of Nursing Knowledge*. London: Routledge.

Russell, S., Daly, J., Hughes, E., Op't Hoog, C. (2003) Nurses and 'difficult' patients: negotiating non-compliance. *Journal of Advanced Nursing*, **43**(3), 281–7.

Scott, H. (2002) Nurses will only get more pay if they take on new roles. *British Journal of Nursing*, **11**(9), 596–7.

Shields, L. & Watson, R. (2007) The demise of nursing in the United Kingdom: a warning for medicine. *Journal of the Royal Society of Medicine*, **100**, 70–4.

Stark, S., Skidmore, D., Warne, T. & Stronach, I. (2002) A survey of 'teamwork' in mental health: is it achievable in practice? *British Journal of Nursing*, **11**(3), 178–86.

Wilhelmsson, S. & Foldevi, M. (2003) Exploring views on Swedish district nurses' prescribing – a focus group study in primary health care. *Journal of Clinical Nursing*, **12**, 643–50.

4

Nurse prescribing experienced

Eleanor Bradley

This chapter focuses on the direct experiences of nurses who successfully completed the prescribing course and set about establishing their prescribing role in practice. The data were derived from postal questionnaires and semi-structured in-depth interviews conducted with nurses working in different environments, specialities and different team formations. Not all visualised the prescribing role in the same way, and this appears to have been dictated by their own perceptions of what they understood non-medical prescribing to be, what their employers expected of them on completion of the course and what they were permitted to do in the services in which they worked. Some had elected to combine supplementary and independent prescribing, while others were working exclusively as either supplementary or as independent prescribers. Approximately a third of the sample anticipated that prescribing would enable them to develop their practice by managing their own caseloads, initiating new ways of working and running nurse-led clinics; others hoped that prescribing would help them reduce the amount of time patients had to wait to be seen and the bureaucracy that accompanies making appointments.

Starting out as a prescriber: overcoming anxiety

Recognising the many dimensions of nurse prescribing and the multiple ways in which it affected nurses, one nurse commenting on her new role summed it up as 'It's a sort of growing up experience'. Approximately two thirds of the sample who opted to become prescribers had already been 'informally prescribing', or prescribing 'by proxy', for a number of years and felt that they had developed a sound working knowledge of the medicines used within their areas of specialty. They were familiar with the medicines used, these medicines were central to the types of care and treatment they provided and patients were accepting that medicines were either central to their treatment or were combined with other forms of nursing care. These nurses also had considerable experience of discussing medicines with doctors and of explaining to service users why certain drugs were being prescribed and what effects they might have on the service users' health. Despite this in-depth knowledge and experience, actually writing their first prescription independently triggered much soul searching. The extent to which they felt 'scared and anxious about making a decision to prescribe' far exceeded their expectations. Having advised countless doctors and patients in the past, having read extensively about these medicines and being convinced that these were the best treatments for patients, one respondent stated, 'I was overcome with overwhelming uncertainty and the thought that I was being asked to prescribe and take responsibility for my actions almost paralysed me'. Nurses acknowledged that giving advice was quite different from taking responsibility for prescribing, and at least a quarter of the sample put off writing their first prescription until 'a modicum, of composure had been restored and a degree of confidence had returned'. Some nurses wrote their first prescription several times on a piece of a paper, checking and re-checking it before eventually writing it out formally for the service user. Such was the doubt that befell some nurses that, in the words of one nurse, 'I have seen the drug written down millions of times, I have seen it prescribed by doctors and I have discussed it several times with doctors and patients, but when I wrote it down it did not look right'. Some described how their hands trembled, while others were assailed by thoughts of awful consequences that could ensue from the act of writing a prescription. One nurse commented that it felt 'as if all the insecurities within nursing arose in me at that moment'.

A common theme among the recently qualified nurse prescribers was a heightened sense of awareness of the responsibility and accountability that came with prescribing as an autonomous practitioner. Some anxiety centred on the awareness that even routine prescriptions have the potential for adverse effects. Prescribing independently also placed pressure on nurses to make the final decisions about medication, whether this be starting a new course of medication, changing to a different medicine or altering the dose of one previously prescribed. Being able to write a prescription without having it authorised by a medical prescriber meant that nurses lost their 'safety net'. When they were prescribing 'by proxy' – advising doctors about the prescription that should be written – the final responsibility still lay ultimately with the doctor, thus relieving nurses of the burden of responsibility. Some nurses expressed surprise at how dependent they had unconsciously become on doctors to check the justification for the prescription. Although nurse prescribers are still encouraged to discuss prescribing decisions with medical colleagues and other appropriate team members such as pharmacists, prescribing independently removes the requirement that this must happen before a prescription is issued. In the absence of having to refer their decisions to a second opinion, nurses acknowledged that they subjected their actions to intense scrutiny, checking the prescriptions they had written and questioning their rationale for issuing a prescription in the first place. In the minds of some it was as if they felt that nursing interventions had been subverted, or were found to be redundant, and that they were instrumental in privileging medicines over other types of care and treatment. Perhaps the degree of apprehension expressed by the nurses was due largely to the conditions under which they were asked to reflect honestly on how they felt, as opposed to getting on with the job. It is possible that some of the prescribers dealt with their anxieties without recourse to anyone else for assistance. Though a degree of caution is desirable, and necessary, to ensure that the level of drug errors reduce, it is possible nevertheless, that an inordinate level of stress could render nurses so insecure that they opt not to prescribe at all.

While all the interviewees eventually came to terms with their initial anxieties, some were surprised by the intensity of feeling that adopting the role induced in them. It appears to have been assumed on the parts of employers and lecturers that because nurses manage anxieties in others, they could manage it in themselves. The emphasis in lectures was very much on the imparting of information with little attention being devoted to the emotional dimension of putting prescribing into practice. In a climate where new roles are being created and the expectation is that health professionals will adapt, it is possible that the supportive environment which may have existed in the past no longer exists. Perhaps some of the concern expressed by these nurses maybe due to the increased litigation that now prevails in healthcare. As one acute care nurse prescriber pointed out, 'the more our role expands, the more scope there is for me to be sued'.

While most nurse prescribers experienced some apprehension on writing their first prescription, those working in certain specialities appeared more vulnerable, particularly those working in children's services. Calculating the dose of medicines appropriate for a child, being aware of the potential long-term side effects, and ensuring collaboration with parents were some of the concerns mentioned. Other 'scary' specialty areas in relation to prescribing included mental health care, care of older adults and learning disability services. Nurses who are prescribing in these areas are rarely prescribing for one condition in isolation; their clients tend to present with multiple problems, some of which will be treated while others may be ignored or referred to other practitioners. For example, in mental health, many service users have physical conditions, some of which may aggravate their mental health problems and need to be taken into consideration in choosing medication. In the area of learning disabilities, there are no medicines specifically licensed for the treatment of what is known as 'learning disability', although the various conditions that service users may suffer from are similar to those of the general population. Although nurse prescribers are responsible for ensuring that they remain within their scope of practice, this scope may, in fact, be very wide. It was clear that nurse prescribers who experienced difficulties in setting their boundaries for prescribing were more subject to anxiety about their new role than those with a more closely defined remit.

In terms of how the role was experienced in practice, there was a clear distinction between nurses who elected to work as supplementary prescribers and those who became independent prescribers. Devising a clinical management plan (CMP), which all supplementary prescribers were expected to do, was time-consuming but had a number of beneficial effects. Because the CMP required formal input and agreement from a medical practitioner and a patient, it reduced the responsibility that some nurses felt about their prescribing decisions. Collaborating with a medical prescriber, in particular, reassured them that they were not being asked to assume ultimate responsibility for what was prescribed. Even though they felt that the CMP reduced their prescribing autonomy, their anxiety about prescribing was reduced far more than it would have been had they been prescribing independently.

Extending the role of nurses into what was once exclusively medical territory has brought to the fore many issues that have rendered the nursing profession insecure over the decades, such as nurses' status in healthcare, the hierarchical nature of healthcare and power relations between doctors and nurses. With the creation of a plethora of new nursing roles, it seems that some nurses, nervous about being asked to do more than they feel capable of, seek continued dependency on doctors while paying lip service to the profession's drive to gain autonomy from them. Although the intended aim of introducing nurse prescribing was to increase service users' access to medicines and to streamline their care, it may well be the case that the unintended aim was to increase the professional standing of nurses within the National Health Service (NHS). Despite many attempts over the history of the NHS to make nurses less dependent on doctors, nurse prescribing may be the vehicle through which it is finally achieved. As well as having benefits for patients, it may also have many benefits for nurses, chief of which is that they can do far more than they have traditionally been allowed.

Despite all these reservations, the majority of nurses felt relief and pride when they were finally able to sign their own prescriptions. Becoming a nurse prescriber legitimised a role they had long been acting out informally. As prescribers, the nurses enjoyed additional status and the formal acknowledgement of their expertise in relation to medicines. Nonetheless, it took some nurses a long time to adjust to their new roles, and there were instances cited of how they 'forgot' that they could sign their own prescriptions and instead continued to ask doctors to sign them.

Starting out as a prescriber: giving information and advice

There was general agreement amongst the nurses that the prescribing course had helped them to become more knowledgeable about prescribing and the medicines with which they were working. The course had helped them to reflect on the ways in which they had previously made decisions about prescribing. They had become far more aware of the complexity of prescribing, of the multiplicity of factors that should influence prescribing decisions and the amount of knowledge required before a prescribing decision could safely be made. Post-qualification, the nurses felt that they would be much more informative and candid in giving advice to service users and colleagues than they would have been prior to doing the course. Some commented that they regarded advice giving to be a form of prescribing, particularly when service users could buy medicines over the counter on their recommendation. They now understood the need to be very clear about what they were saying to service users because they were aware that their words might influence whether medicines were taken and whether clients would be able to cope with adverse side effects. The course had also helped the nurses to appreciate why doctors were so cautious about signing prescriptions for service users that they had not seen or diagnosed themselves.

The nurses felt that, as prescribers, they were more likely to discuss the impact of medicines with service users than they had been before. They wanted to find out whether the medicine they had prescribed had had the desired effect and been acceptable to the patient. They felt they had become more attentive to what service users were saying about their conditions, even when they were not visiting them for the specific purpose of reviewing their medication. The nurses were quite sure that prescribing had encouraged them to spend more time discussing and evaluating the impact of prescribed medication with their service users with a view to addressing issues around adherence to treatment regimes.

Nurses recognised that prescribing brings with it a responsibility to keep their pharmacological knowledge up to date post-qualification. When nurses occupied leadership roles within teams which included more junior nurse prescribers, they felt the need to keep up to date particularly strongly so that they did not 'lag behind'. It is reassuring that the nurses were so aware of the need to keep their prescribing knowledge current because the prescribing course is generic in content, and participants must take responsibility for ensuring that they develop the specific knowledge required in their specialty areas. Employer organisations must give their nurse prescribers the time and opportunity to maintain their knowledge and develop their practice. For most of the nurses interviewed, organisational support was not as forthcoming as they would have liked it to be.

Becoming confident and competent

The prescribing was not designed to provide nurses with information specific to their specialty areas, and successful completion of the course was certainly not intended to signal the end of nurses' training in prescribing. Instead, the course provides the basics of prescribing upon which nurses can build when prescribing in their specialty areas. Some nurses were content that the prescribing course provided a starting point for their practice, but others felt that the information and knowledge gained from the course served only to highlight their ignorance around prescribing and medication and to indicate whole new areas of knowledge that they needed to gain before they could feel confident starting to prescribe. As one nurse commented about his experiences since qualifying, 'it's almost like the more you find out, the more you realise what you don't know or what you still need to know'. Kruger and Dunning (1999) discuss 'not knowing what you don't know' and explain that incompetence in a particular task makes it impossible to evaluate how successfully the task has been achieved. Individuals who lack competence lack the self-monitoring skills necessary to judge their competence and so cannot tell when they make an error. They may leave others with the mistaken impression that they are doing 'just fine'. Some of the nurses described how, prior to doing the prescribing course, they had been under the false impression that they had been making good prescribing decisions. Only after training and gaining new knowledge did they become aware of, and evaluate, their previous incompetence.

The realisation that they were not as competent as they had previously thought may come as a blow to nurses' confidence and cause them to identify areas in which they require further training before they feel competent to start prescribing. However, this could become an endless circle of identifying areas in which knowledge is not complete, seeking further training and then identifying yet new areas that need strengthening. While it is important that nurses who opt to prescribe feel confident in their knowledge, they also need to learn how to maximise in their practice the knowledge they have and to get support on the job to help them improve. Many nurses begin their prescribing careers by prescribing only those medicines with which they are very familiar and for service users they know well. The prescribing role should evolve at its own pace rather than being forced to occur too quickly. Taking things slowly serves to reassure other prescribing professionals that nurses can limit their prescribing practice to those areas in which they have manifest knowledge and allows the nurses time to expand the scope of their practice as their knowledge grows.

As new prescribers, nurses described feeling acutely aware that they must keep within their competencies. There was a strong feeling that legislation to 'open up' the British National Formulary (BNF) to nurses, permitting them to prescribe from almost the same range of medicines as doctors, should not encourage them to start prescribing outside their speciality areas. Nonetheless, the fact that they had been given access to the full range of medicines was cautiously welcomed by most nurses and regarded as acknowledgement of their status as autonomous practitioners. As long as extended independent and supplementary prescribing remains new to nurses, it is likely that they will be restrained in using their prescribing rights.

Prescribing decision making

Despite increased autonomy, the nurses continued to favour discussing prescribing decisions with other prescribing team members. They also consulted with service users and looked up the relevant research evidence. The degree of collaboration depends on the configuration of teams within which nurse prescribers are working. Large teams increase access to doctors and make collaboration easier than for nurse prescribers working in isolation across a community setting. In some teams, collaboration between nurse and doctor remains the norm before any prescribing decisions are made, and this is to be commended. The prescribing course requires that nurses have a medical mentor to help them develop their prescribing role in practice. Post-qualification, the role of mentors is less formal, but many nurses continue to turn to them for advice. In the best-case scenario, the medical mentors are an invaluable resource, and some nurses reported that medical colleagues had become more willing to discuss prescribing decisions with them once they were qualified as prescribers and that they themselves have become more confident to engage in such discussions. On the other hand, some had insufficient confidence to contest the prescribing decisions of their medical colleagues. When nurses are able to prescribe only within a supplementary prescribing model, they are wholly reliant on the support of their medical prescriber before they can put a prescribing plan into place, and this unequal relationship discourages them from challenging prescribing decisions. The current reliance on medical prescribers to assume the role of the mentor/clinical tutor whilst the nurse is taking the prescribing qualification reinforces traditional hierarchies. The nurse depends on the medical mentor 'signing off' his or her capability to prescribe and is thus unlikely to challenge the mentor's prescribing decisions. One way of addressing this problem is for experienced nurse prescribers to take on the role of mentors/clinical tutors. This will assist in dismantling the hierarchical structure of healthcare that often stands in the way of true collaboration.

Prescribing decisions are heavily influenced by directions from consultant colleagues, Trust policies, National Institute for Clinical Excellence (NICE) guidelines and drug budgets. Decisions about which medicines to use must be firmly grounded in up-to-date evidence. However, in some specialty areas, such as paediatric dermatology, there is currently a lack of evidence to assist prescribing decisions. In such instances, nurse prescribers need to be led by service user preference rather than prescribing tradition. As teams come to include new prescribers, prescribing can be viewed from new perspectives, and such a shift in the status quo is to be embraced rather than resisted. This study has suggested that nurses are keen to consult and agree with their service users prior to selecting medication. When medication is selected on the basis of service user preference, it is more likely that concordance with treatment regimes will be achieved.

Nurses acknowledge that prescribing decisions can be made out of habit or familiarity with a particular medication. The art of prescribing lies in the ability to update prescribing choices through critical appraisal of past decision making and service user feedback. Discussion and debate with prescribing colleagues is part of ensuring that prescribing does not fall into habitual patterns, although some prescribers may feel threatened by such an open approach to prescribing practice. When nurses were observing medical prescribing, they felt that decisions were often made in the absence of a formal rationale or structured decision-making process. It was prescribers' personal preferences for treatment choices that were reflected in the decisions they made about prescribing. It may be that prescribing preferences are formed during training by observing the practice of prescribing mentors. However, the opposite should be the case, with nurse prescribers presenting an opportunity for doctors to engage in a critical reflective process around their prescribing and to consider a nursing perspective gained from experience in different specialties. The basis of mentoring should be discussion between doctors and nurses about treatment choices and prescribing options.

Making a prescribing decision is not always about deciding which is the best prescription to write; it is sometimes about whether to prescribe at all. Prescribers who stem from a nursing rather than a medical background may be more inclined to consider non-pharmacological options. Over the past two decades, nurse training has increasingly transmitted a psychosocial approach to care. Today's nurses may therefore be more attuned to non-pharmacological therapeutic approaches and likely to employ these as their first-line approach to care. Nurses who see their service users in the community also have the advantage of being able to consider the social context in which service users are managing their condition and receiving treatment. This gives them the opportunity to work more holistically with service users than doctors do, and a holistic approach should inform their prescribing decisions. As one nurse noted, 'the difference between medical and nurse prescribing is that the medical role is very focussed and specific. Doctors are dealing with symptoms that are being reported at a specific time in a fixed location, whereas, in nursing, service users are seen in a variety of situations and settings and the nurse has to make sense of reported symptoms and experiences that will be affected by these different situations'. Even where nurses are seeing their service users in situations akin to the medical consultation, such as practice nurses working in general practitioner (GP) practices, the enhanced communication that is possible between nurse and service user (as reported in many studies, including Luker, 1997) and the longer appointment times that some nurses have retained encourage users to share their thoughts and feelings with the nurse. This will help nurses make prescribing decisions that 'fit' with the service user.

It appears from this study, however, that some nurses feel pressured always to prescribe because prescribing is what they have trained to do. If they are not prescribing, how can they justify becoming a nurse prescriber? This type of pressure emanates from a misunderstanding of the nurse prescribing role. Although nurse prescribers are able to prescribe, their non-prescribing colleagues should not see them solely as 'the prescribing nurse'. They must not be regarded as an easy way of accessing prescribed medication by service users or team members, and they should be prescribing only for service users whom they have seen.

Clinical management plans

Supplementary prescribers are unable to prescribe without a clinical management plan (CMP). The CMP generated plentiful debate among the nurses consulted for this study. It appears that there is considerable misunderstanding among doctors about the purpose of the CMP, and nurse prescribers need actively to clarify its use. There is potential for abuse of the CMP, with some plans being used in ways that resemble standardised Patient Group Directives (PGDs) rather than individualised care plans. We were told of instances when plans were drawn up by nurses and signed off by medical prescribers rather than being discussed and written collaboratively. Used in this way, the CMP is simply another manifestation of nurses prescribing 'by proxy' rather than a tool for carefully designed treatment interventions. CMPs are employed variously in different practice settings, and this increases nurses' difficulties in explaining their purpose to doctors and also to service users. One nurse prescriber had found it helpful to produce a leaflet that explained CMPs to service users. Such a leaflet would also be helpful for prescribing and non-prescribing team members.

Clinical management plans are relatively time-consuming to produce; they have to be negotiated with doctors, written and then discussed with doctors and service users. Nurses commonly have no clerical support in their prescribing role, yet drawing up CMPs involves administrative tasks including writing letters to GPs when changes are made. When a lot of information is required, the limited space available on the CMP has proved problematic, and there is frustration when there is a significant overlap with care plans and other documentation. Some nurses found it useful to integrate their CMPs with case notes to save them constantly having to rewrite information. Reducing the amount of information in the CMP was felt to be helpful for service users who sometimes found it confusing. Opinions on the amount of information that should be included on a CMP were, however, divided. Some nurses felt that they wanted to be very specific so that their prescribing was well defined, while others preferred to include the minimum of information so that their practice could retain an element of flexibility. Nurse prescribers clearly need time to 'get comfortable' with the CMP, questioning and adapting the structure of the pro formas, looking at how much detail should be included. One useful way of managing

CMPs in practice appears to be by via a 'generic' CMP, which is then tailored to individual patients.

The settings in which CMPs are used strongly influence how successfully they are implemented. Nurses working across community settings in teams without any full-time medical support experienced significant delays in getting changes to CMPs agreed. Yet it is precisely these nurses who need to be able to use their prescribing role efficiently so that they can offer their service users appropriate, timely and flexible care. Equally challenging was getting a CMP confirmed when nurses were working alongside a large number of medical prescribers, particularly if each doctor had a different view of the role of the supplementary prescriber and how CMPs should be put together to support this role. The time spent negotiating and preparing CMPs may influence some doctors not to support supplementary prescribing, and some nurses who are able to prescribe only as supplementary prescribers may decide to revert to their previous practice of prescribing 'by proxy' rather than going to the trouble of putting a CMP in place to enable them to prescribe directly.

The nurses welcomed the fact that the CMP obliges nurses and doctors to consider carefully all possible implications of the chosen medication and includes alternatives to avoid a new plan having to be drawn up at a later date. The CMP was also thought to be helpful in making prescribing decisions transparent to service users who have access to their own CMPs. Many of the nurse prescribers found that the plan was helpful when they qualified as prescribers because it provides a helpful structure to guide them in thinking through their prescribing, thereby alleviating some of the anxiety they felt when they were first making prescribing decisions. Even nurses who were predominantly prescribing independently used the CMP to guide their decision making and reassure them about the safety of what they were doing. Some nurses felt frustrated that they had to review their CMPs with the medical prescriber on a 3-monthly basis when they could have taken responsibility for doing this themselves. However, the nurses also acknowledged that regular review benefited service users.

'Knowing' the service user

It has been well documented that service users find it easier to talk to nurses and feel less pressured than with doctors; they therefore tend to ask more questions and reveal more about their problems (Luker *et al.*, 1997; Davis & Hemingway, 2003; Hem & Heggen, 2003). Because nurses have traditionally had more time to spend with service users, there is more opportunity for users to mention co-existing conditions and for nurses to discuss treatments and their potential side effects in detail. These factors increase service users' satisfaction with the care they receive (Venning *et al.*, 2000). Even in GP surgeries, where nurses have the same appointment times as doctors, users still report that they feel the nurse has more time for their consultation. Nurses felt that their rapport with service users meant that users were able to ask 'silly' questions, and users described themselves as being more honest when answering questions about their health. Some service users felt that they would go and see the nurse about symptoms that they wouldn't 'worry the doctor' about. Nurses are more likely to remain involved in the care of service users diagnosed with chronic conditions than doctors, whose involvement may be more transient. Certainly nurses reported that service users feel that their nurse knows them better than their doctor and that this, coupled with more frequent contact, enables nurses to keep a careful eye on medication.

In mental health nursing, it is particularly important that prescribing professionals have the opportunity to get to know their service users, who may find it difficult to communicate their experiences, may interpret their symptoms differently from health professionals, may disagree with the diagnosis, may be reluctant to take prescribed medication and may have a number of co-existing physical conditions. The mental health nurses in this study felt that doctors saw only a 'snapshot' of the service user, whereas they often had the opportunity to get to know the users over a long period of time and visit them in various settings, including their home environment. 'Knowing' the service user was perceived to influence decision making about treatments and medication. Some nurses gathered information about the impact treatment was having on the user by talking to carers and family members as well as the service user, and it was felt that this improved prescribing accuracy. For nurses working with service users diagnosed with learning disabilities, knowledge of the family was felt to be essential to understanding and communicating with the service users about their medications. Nurses were aware of the temptation in the area of learning disabilities to see only problem behaviours and medicate them. However, by spending time with and observing the users and their families, they felt more able to challenge inappropriate prescribing decisions and over-medication. Mental health nurses working in GP practices felt that their service users regarded them as the 'experts' in mental health medication. In some cases, users did not feel that they had been asked by their doctors about their experiences of medication and so particularly appreciated the opportunity to discuss these with their nurse.

Benefits of nurse prescribing

The nurses saw their ability to provide service users with a complete package of care – by their assuming responsibility for assessing, prescribing, monitoring and reviewing medication – as highly beneficial to users. They were able to increase the efficiency with which service users had their medication initiated or altered, and this speed of response was particularly appreciated by users and their families during a crisis. Nurse prescribing was regarded as very responsive to service users' needs because nurses were more accessible than doctors. When nurses were acting as supplementary prescribers, the CMP was seen to encourage more regular review of medication than had previously been the case, and this was felt to assist in preventing crises from happening in the first place.

Nurses felt that they now gave more time to listening to service users describing their symptoms, medication experiences and preferences now that they were able to write the prescription themselves. When they had been prescribing 'by proxy', they had spent more of their time thinking about how they were going to get their prescriptions signed than listening to service users' concerns. Nurse prescribers believed that they were good at involving users in prescribing decisions and providing them with information and education about their medication. At a time when offering choice to service users is seen as a priority in healthcare, having a nurse prescriber within the healthcare team was felt to be a means of offering service users a choice of prescriber.

The nurses felt that their practice had been enhanced as a consequence of prescribing. Specifically, they felt able to offer a more holistic approach to care as a result of their prescribing training, which had enhanced their awareness of many types of interventions.

The nurses felt that they had gained personally from becoming prescribers. They enjoyed increased self-esteem and job satisfaction as well as a satisfaction in providing enhanced patient care. They felt more educated about medication in general and more confident in communicating this information to service users and carers. They also felt that their ability to communicate with other prescribers about medication, including doctors, had improved and that this, in turn, had increased the potential for collaborative activities within and across healthcare teams. These benefits were realised even by those nurse prescribers who had not prescribed in practice. Nurse prescribers were regarded as 'experts' in medication in their specialty areas and were sought out by colleagues for information about medicines and prescribing. This could be challenging for the nurses but ensured that they kept up to date and motivated them to develop their knowledge further. The nurses felt that their increased knowledge was reflected in an increase in the knowledge of service users because nurses were spending more time giving them information and educating them about their conditions, as well as looking in more detail at the impact that medication might have. Taking the prescribing course with a range of people from different specialities had encouraged the nurses to develop their knowledge in other areas. One mental health nurse commented that she was now far better informed about the physical problems that her service users might experience and was paying more attention to assessment of physical well-being.

Increased knowledge about medicines had encouraged some nurses to become more proactive in the interests of their service users. They were more willing to check prescriptions written by doctors and more confident challenging prescribing decisions. As team members, nurse prescribers felt they took pressure off doctors by decreasing their workload, reducing waiting times for service users and being able to sign prescriptions.

Barriers to prescribing

Fifty per cent of the nurses we consulted felt that there had been barriers to overcome before they could start prescribing. Many barriers were organisational, with some workplaces failing to put the relevant systems and policies in place to support nurse prescribing in practice. The early nurse prescribers (the 'pioneers') played a key role in dismantling these barriers; indeed, the development of appropriate systems and policies was deemed to be a major part of the nurse prescribers' role post-qualification (see Chapter 3 for more discussion of the 'pioneers'). Early cohorts of nurse prescribers working in community mental health teams attached to GP surgeries spent much time post-qualification trying to organise service level agreements across different organisations to enable them to gain access to prescribing pads. This proved an extremely tortuous process. Some of the pioneers felt that dismantling organisational barriers was beyond their remit and simply opted not to put their prescribing qualification into practice. Further, barriers to practice still remain, even in those organisations where nurses have been prescribing since 2003. It was not unusual for nurses in our study to report waiting between 9 and 12 months to receive a prescribing pad. Many are unable to access electronic prescribing systems in their workplaces, forcing them to handwrite prescriptions and increasing the amount of administration associated with prescribing. Some nurses struggle to gain access to a budget for prescribing and have to spend time finding out from their employer Trusts which budget they should be using. Healthcare organisations need a clear strategy for nurse prescribing because nurses can lose the motivation to prescribe if they are unable to use their skills soon after qualification. Some of the pioneers opted not to prescribe because they felt they had lost their confidence whilst waiting for permission to start practising. This phenomenon has been reported in the literature (Otway, 2001).

Difficulties with implementation

Not all barriers to prescribing are organisational. Some nurses find it difficult to decide how to implement their new prescribing role in practice. Nurses in the first cohorts to undertake the prescribing course were unclear about the types of prescribing that they would be able to engage in post-qualification. Some did not realise until they started the course that they would not be able to prescribe independently in their specialty areas. Their teams were not prepared for the fact that the nurse would be a *supplementary* prescriber. Because supplementary prescribing requires a high degree of collaboration and support, team members must have a good understanding of what is involved, of how working with a supplementary prescriber might have an impact on their roles and of the practical issues surrounding the CMPs. The time it takes to prescribe as a supplementary prescriber is a barrier when nurses do not have the time to complete CMPs and experience difficulty in finding supportive doctors who are prepared to collaborate on the paperwork. In many cases nurses found it was quicker to request a prescription from a doctor than to draw up a CMP.

Nurses who are going to be the first nurse prescribers in their teams would benefit from guidance at an early stage of the prescribing course about how to implement their prescribing role. The course attracts a wide range of nurses from different workplaces and specialties and so provides a valuable opportunity to discuss the varying ways in which prescribing can be put into practice. Discussion of CMPs and their use in different settings would be particularly helpful for nurses intending to operate as supplementary prescribers within hospital settings where CMPs may have to be drawn up for groups of patients rather than individually. Some nurses may need to set up nurse-led clinics in order to utilise their prescribing role, and this requires time and organisational and team support.

Support and remuneration

The anxiety that nurses feel about their prescribing role has already been highlighted. Nurses need to feel encouraged to prescribe and need access to formal and informal support from both prescribing and non-prescribing team members. Medical colleagues' perceived lack of enthusiasm for non-medical prescribing undermines nurses' confidence and can delay the implementation of prescribing in practice. Some doctors are unclear about the purpose and potential of the CMP and, where difficulties have been experienced previously with nurse prescribing, may be cautious about introducing new nurse prescribers to their teams. They may also be concerned that nurses will increase their prescribing costs. Nurses need to spend time explaining their prescribing role to professionals, especially doctors and pharmacists, across the teams, and how they hope to implement prescribing. Their aim should be to alleviate concerns and discuss how they see non-medical prescribing influencing service development.

Mentors are a principal source of support for many nurse prescribers; however, access to them is dependent on the setting in which the nurses are working. In hospitals or GP surgeries, nurses tend to work in close proximity to their medical mentors and other medical colleagues. Arranging formal sessions to discuss prescribing issues is unnecessary; the nurse can 'drop in' to see the doctor. However, nurses working across community settings or within teams that do not have full-time medical members have to rely on organised sessions that may be less frequent and less timely. While lack of access to medical support can be a barrier to prescribing practice, easy access and regular contact with medical prescribers can equally be a problem. If nurses work closely with doctors, there is the temptation to forego the responsibility of writing their own prescriptions and continue to prescribe by proxy in the traditional manner.

Many nurses feel aggrieved that they receive little remuneration for obtaining their prescribing qualification. The training course is intensive and challenging, particularly for nurses who have not studied in an academic environment for a number of years. Nurses were disappointed that having a prescribing qualification was not recognised in the *Agenda for Change* banding exercise in the UK. Some nurses feel that prescribing is one more role being added to an already onerous job, a role that significantly increases their responsibility, and yet which attracts no financial reward. In an increasingly difficult financial climate, it is unlikely that the prescribing qualification will attract monetary recognition. To compensate, organisational recognition in the form of support for ongoing training and education is essential to encourage nurses to take up this new role and feel positively about it.

Role change and service development

For some nurses, the prescribing qualification is a step in their career development. Having attained it, some are promoted, or experience further role changes that may render prescribing unnecessary because they no longer have a clinical role or have a vastly reduced one. Increasingly, nurses take the prescribing qualification because it is a requirement of either another course such as an M.Sc. in advanced practice or a new job. The prescribing qualification is increasingly unlikely to be an end in itself, and the intentions of students taking the course may be even more diverse than those of the nurse prescribing pioneers who saw prescribing as a means of developing their practice. Nurse educators delivering the prescribing course will need to be aware of the range of students' motivation for undertaking training and consider how prescribing relates to a wide range of roles and many different settings (Bradley *et al.*, 2006). They are also likely to find themselves teaching ever more highly educated cohorts of nurses.

For some nurses, the primary aim of becoming a nurse prescriber was to develop a clinical practice; however, on qualification, they found that this would be possible only if they undertook significant service development. Some nurses opted to prescribe because they wanted to establish nurse-led clinics. Unfortunately, the money to do this was not in place before the nurse started training, and later bids proved unsuccessful. If service development was financially impossible, nurses were then unable to utilise their prescribing. Such a situation is de-motivating and undermines aspirations to design innovative new services.

REFERENCES

Bradley, E. J., Blackshaw, C. & Nolan, P. (2006) Nurse lecturers' observations on aspects of nurse prescribing training. *Nurse Education Today*, **26**, 538–44.

Davis, J. & Hemingway, S. (2003) Supplementary prescribing in mental health nursing. *Nursing Times*, **99**(32), 28–30.

Hem, M. H., & Heggen, K. (2003) Being professional and being human: one nurse's relationship with a psychiatric patient. *Journal of Advanced Nursing*, **43**(1), 101–8.

Kruger, J. & Dunning, D. (1999) Unskilled and unaware of it. *Journal of Personality and Social Psychology*, **77**(6), 1121–34.

Luker, K. (1997) *Evaluation of Nurse Prescribing. Final Report.* Liverpool: University of Liverpool and University of York.

Luker, K. A., Austin, L., Hogg, C., Ferguson, B. & Smith K. (1997) Nurse prescribing: the views of nurses and other health care professionals. *British Journal of Community Nursing*, **2**(2), 69–74.

Otway, C. (2001) Informal peer support: a key to success for nurse prescribers. *British Journal of Community Nursing*, **6**, 586–91.

Venning, P., Durie, A., Roland, M., Roberts, C. & Leese, B. (2000) Randomised controlled trial comparing cost-effectiveness of general practitioners and nurse practitioners in primary care. *British Medical Journal*, **320**, 1048–53.

Nurse prescribing observed

Eleanor Bradley, Peter Nolan and Tanvir Rana

Unlike other prescribers who work solely in private practice, the majority of nurses do not work in isolation; instead, they work in a variety of teams and organisations. To implement non-medical prescribing successfully, it goes without saying that the prescribers need to be competent, confident and adaptable. In addition, there are other important factors that will influence the success of this new venture. These include the composition of the team in which nurses are working, the quality of communication within the team and the extent to which each member understands the role of other members. New ways of working require professionals to be open to change and rethink professional boundaries because change involves many more than those charged with initiating it. There must be clear benefits to having a nurse prescriber within the team, and all team members much be prepared to support him or her. If teams do not understand the role or, worse, feel that the role has been imposed on them, it is highly likely that disillusionment and dysfunctionality will arise. Equally, the attitudes of service users towards nurses' prescribing role and their understanding of it are critical because the way in which they engage with nurse prescribers will determine whether the anticipated benefits of nurse prescribing are realised or not.

This chapter is based on the findings of three studies which focused on service users' experiences of nurse prescribing, the attitudes and experiences of healthcare team members towards nurse prescribing and, finally, the views of doctors. In-depth interviews were conducted with 10 service users. Two of these suffered from asthma, two had diabetes, three had enduring mental health problems and three suffered from chronic pain. At the time of the interviews, all were receiving care and treatment from nurse prescribers. The interviewees were selected on the basis that their conditions had persisted for at least 10 years, that they had received treatment from various services and from personnel both inside and outside the National Health Service (NHS) and that they were generally well informed about their health problems and needs. Eight were currently involved in self-help groups, and five had carers who were part of a support network for those caring for people with conditions similar to their own. All 10 regularly consulted the Internet and used websites which they believed to give authoritative, up-to-date advice.

Service user perspectives

Nurse prescribers had commonly become involved with the service users following a hospital stay. Some had been referred to a nurse prescriber by their general practitioner (GP), who had told them that the nurse prescribers were 'specialists' in caring for people with their particular chronic condition and that they would therefore be able to provide better information and care than they, the GPs, could as 'generalists'.

Stigma

Many of the interviewees felt that they were stigmatised by health professionals as a result of their diagnoses, particularly when their condition could be attributed in part to lifestyle choices such as diet or smoking.

Profiles of interviewees X and Y

Participant X has a weight problem. This is the result of taking prescribed steroids for a condition co-existing with her diabetes. She finds it stressful to attend outpatients' appointments at the local hospital because she has overheard negative comments about her weight from nursing and medical staff and finds these both hurtful and uninformed. Her nurse prescriber is, however, aware of her struggle with her weight and understands the factors aggravating it. She feels that doctors make judgements about her condition before she has even sat down but that her nurse prescriber places her weight problem in context.

Participant Y has asthma and is aware that smoking aggravates her condition. When she attended the hospital, she found it difficult to admit to hospital staff that she was a smoker because she felt that she would 'be told off'. On being referred to a nurse prescriber, she was initially concerned that the nurse would focus on her smoking habit and be judgemental. However, after seeing the nurse, she felt that he understood the difficulties she had had in attempting to give up smoking. Even though the nurse was keen that she should continue to try to give up, Y felt that his attitude had been far more helpful than that of other healthcare staff and, as a consequence, that his advice was more acceptable.

In both these cases, the nurse prescriber had the opportunity to get to know the service user and to start to understand her lifestyle choices and motivations. Getting to know someone is essential to prevent the recipient of care feeling stigmatised (Hogg & Vaughan, 1995), and nurse prescribers who are working on a long-term basis with their service users have the opportunity to confront their own prejudices and eliminate initial stigmatising responses as they increase their understanding of the complexities of clients' lives. Service users appreciated having the time to explain their struggles to cut out unhealthy behaviours and felt that the nurses were able to provide advice grounded in the context of their real lives. All the respondents indicated that being known, feeling understood and knowing that the person caring for them had their best interests at heart were very important factors in ensuring successful outcomes of care. Research, such as that carried out by Williams and Jones (2006), has found differences in the consulting styles of nurses and doctors and has suggested that nurses' approach to discussing health promotional activities (or 'giving up' unhealthy behaviours) is helpful in identifying a best option for service users' future behaviour (even if they decide not to pursue it). Whereas nurses seek to create an egalitarian relationship with service users, some doctors in the past have tended to espouse the traditional medical model approach in which the doctor knows best and patients should conform (Richman, 2002). In the case of Y, advice about smoking cessation was provided and considered. Even though it did not result in any immediate change, it provided the groundwork for further exploration of healthy behaviours, opening up issues that could be discussed at a later stage when the user might feel more ready to make changes. In the case of service users who have behaviours that are damaging to their health, nurses need to be able to utilise their relationship with them to help reduce or eliminate them. Following service users from the hospital into the community enabled the nurse prescribers to tailor health-promotional advice to the context in which it had to be implemented. As health psychology has repeatedly demonstrated (Billings & Moos, 1981; Miller & Mangan, 1983; Johnson, 1999; Bradley et al., 2001), consideration of clients' motivations, knowledge, 'lay' interpretations and social pressures is important when giving health advice.

Changing behaviour is highly complex, particularly if service users are living in an environment that actively promotes an unhealthy lifestyle (such as living with a partner who smokes or being part of a household accustomed to a high-fat diet). The biggest problem for some people who engage in unhealthy lifestyles is that they do not have regular social contacts with people they respect who could dissuade them from such activities while reinforcing positive behaviour. Nurse prescribers not only require excellent knowledge of the condition they are treating but also need to be able to use techniques for reducing unhealthy behaviours which exacerbate those conditions. Despite this, our survey of nurses in the West Midlands of the UK found that nurses did not consider health promotion to be an important aspect of their prescribing role, nor did they feel that they were in need of any further input on this topic as part of their overall prescribing training (see earlier chapters). While it is possible that nurses feel competent in health promotion because of their extended contact with service users and good knowledge of their specialty areas, a study by Offredy (2002) suggests that nurse practitioners based in GP practices did not always incorporate health education when making decisions on scenarios involving clients with conditions such as pelvic inflammatory disease and hypertension for which health education was clearly indicated. The lack of importance accorded to health promotion by the participants in our study is worrying. Nurses need to be constantly aware of the opportunity they have as prescribers to link information about medicines with information about healthy lifestyles in order to maximise the full therapeutic potential of their new role (Latter *et al.*, 2004). Future research should examine whether nurse prescribers are able to reduce unhealthy behaviours in people diagnosed with long-term, chronic conditions; whether service users are more inclined to discuss these behaviours with nurse prescribers than with their doctor and whether and how nurses and doctors differ in their approach to health promotion.

For the service users diagnosed with mental health problems, knowing and trusting their healthcare professional were particularly important:

Knowing that my Community Psychiatric Nurse is there makes me feel confident about the help that I get and the things that make my life better. (Male diagnosed with mental health problems)

Where service users lack insight into their illness, as can be the case with people diagnosed with mental health problems, having one prescribing professional as a constant feature during episodes of illness could help with the interpretation of symptoms and assist with planning future care and treatment. For the client, having someone known to them confirm that improvement is or will soon be taking place is reassuring at times when they are not able to make an accurate judgement about their own well-being. Respondents with mental health problems did not relate to 'the multi-disciplinary team'; for them, this was meaningless. They liked knowing one person well and had no sense of there being people in the background offering advice and help.

Time to talk

Service users appreciate having time with healthcare professionals, and having that time is perceived as a primary advantage to consulting with a nurse practitioner rather than a GP (Williams & Jones, 2006). GP services in the UK allow patients an average of 4 to 6 minutes with a GP but 10 to 15 minutes with a nurse practitioner (Venning *et al.*, 2000; Williams & Jones, 2006). However, as nurse practitioners increasingly take over work formerly done by GPs, the amount of time that they have to spend with their patients will almost inevitably decrease (Vere-Jones, 2007). Furthermore, in primary care, the number of patients seen determines the income of the practice, so nurses may be required to see the same number of clients as doctors. It is not entirely clear which benefits service users derive from spending time with nurses and whether these are exclusive to nurses or could be achieved by doctors if they had longer consultation times with their clients. The feeling that there is ample time to talk to a nurse about one's health undoubtedly contributes to a sense of being cared for, which is less likely to happen when the consultation appears to be time-limited. Williams and Jones (2006) argue that it is entirely possible that if GPs increased their appointment times, service users' preference for nurse practitioners would decrease. Further, the common assumption that nurses have more effective communication skills than doctors has been challenged (Charles-Jones *et al.*, 2003). Interestingly, the study conducted by Ridsdale *et al.* (1992) into doctors' communication with service users found that an increased amount of time did not necessarily lead to doctors adopting different communication techniques or to greater health gains for clients. Doctors who were good communicators used their skills to a greater degree when they had extra time, but those whose skills were less proficient did not change their communication style when they had more time available. The authors concluded that increased time was a necessary but not sufficient condition to promote better communication techniques during consultations. Research looking at the potential benefits of non-medical prescribing still needs to ascertain whether nurses do provide better information than doctors about conditions and treatments when prescribing or whether the patient's satisfaction with nurse prescribers is reliant on their ongoing, sometimes long-standing relationship with the nurse.

The service users who participated in our study felt that the doctors they saw were busy and very focused on time keeping during appointments. With nurse prescribers, on the other hand, service users felt that they had more time to discuss their problems and symptoms:

I find my GP a little difficult to talk to and always have the sense that they are 'watching the clock'. With the specialist nurse (prescriber) I feel more relaxed; the nurse has more time to spend talking to me and listens to me. (Female, diagnosed with asthma)

A major thing I noticed was she gave me plenty of time and information. Everything was explained, what the blood tests were for, very thorough, very reassuring. She never struck me as being overly busy to the point that I was asked to leave. That contrasted very strongly with doctors who were always keen to move on to the next patient. (Female, diagnosed with arthritis)

A sense of pressure of time at the GP surgery affected service users' decisions about what to 'bother' their doctor with, feeling that anything 'minor' should be dealt with by a nurse and only more serious issues should be kept for the doctor. Building a rapport with the prescribing professional was felt to be important to the outcome of appointments:

The good listeners know you, they are interested in getting to know you better. When you go regularly, they get to know you and you can tell the good ones from the not so good ones. Being listened to and feeling understood improves whatever treatment they provide. (Female, diagnosed with mental health problems)

The importance of being listened to was regarded as highly as being prescribed the right medicine. In a time-pressured consultation, service users felt that they had no time to discuss the context within which they were managing their conditions, how they felt about their prescribed medication and what treatments they would prefer or to find out about non-pharmacological options. Under such circumstances, they felt that doctors were making decisions about treatment without having all the information they needed and ran the risk of taking decisions viewed by the service user as inappropriate or irrelevant. The consequences of this are evident in literature, which suggests that the numbers of people who never cash in their scripts ranges from 14.5% (Beardon *et al.*, 1993) to 25% (Rashid, 1982), and up to half of all prescribed drugs are not taken (Pearce, 2003). Drugs wastage is a significant cost for the NHS in England, with at least £100 million worth of medicines returned unused per year (National Audit Office, 2007). This figure is believed to significantly underestimate the actual cost of drugs wastage, with the Department of Health (DoH) estimating that 10% of all drugs taken are wasted – adding up to £800 million worth of drugs per year (DoH, 2004). The service users taking part in our study regularly asked themselves a series of questions about their medication, including:

- *What side effects can I expect?*
- *What will happen to me if I change my medication several times?*
- *What do I do if the drug doesn't suit me?*
- *If the medication doesn't work, does that mean my illness is worse than I thought, or worse than anybody else's?*
- *How long will I be expected to take the medication?*
- *Will there be any interactions between the drugs I am taking?*

Early experiences of taking prescribed medication were important in influencing attitudes towards future pharmacological intervention:

When I first started taking medication, I was very anti-tablets, but over time I have come to rely on medicines. Now I believe if I stop taking medication, I would relapse almost immediately. The reason why I believe in medicines is that I became convinced that the tablet I took brought me back to normality. I attributed that to taking medication. (Male, diagnosed with mental health problems)

Nurse prescribers, particularly those working across the community setting, currently have more time to listen to service users:

I have longer for consultations with my nurse prescriber and I discuss all aspects of my life and not just my problems. What I appreciate most is that it's not just how I feel at that moment on that particular day, I can talk about how I am feeling over a period of time. (Female, diagnosed with mental health problems)

As well as affecting service user satisfaction, extra time should enable nurses to gather more information to guide their prescribing decisions and to discuss those decisions with service users before issuing a prescription. At the moment, nurse prescribers are in an excellent position to enhance service user satisfaction with care, reduce the costs associated with inappropriate prescribing and tackle issues associated with adherence.

The nurse prescriber was commonly the only professional who remained involved with the care of the service user over a long period. This was very much appreciated by the interviewees in our study, who did not have to waste time at appointments explaining the background to their condition – their symptoms and what made them worse – to professionals who had never seen them before. Nurse prescribers could tailor their appointments to their immediate concerns and recent developments in their medical and personal circumstances. Especially in the early stages of treatment, nurses gave service users the time to talk in general about their understanding of their diagnosis, and consider how they felt about treatment. This was important because service users with little experience of medication or familiarity with their diagnosis did not always know what questions to ask:

At the time, I did not know what to expect and I was not able to say whether the treatment was successful or not. The medication was [an anti-depressant] and I was very scared of taking it. I did not know what information I needed. (Female, diagnosed with mental health problems)

Having more time allowed nurses to attend to the complexity of service users' lives and offer non-pharmacological approaches to treatment (Williams & Jones, 2006). People with health problems need time to explore how their difficulties are affecting all aspects of their being and to examine how they can be active in their own treatment, thereby ensuring that whatever treatment is recommended meets their expectations.

Concordance

Service users often find it difficult to take their medication as prescribed, particularly when they are suffering from a number of conditions and have a complex medication regimen. It is common for people to alter the way in which they take their medicines according to the side effects they are experiencing and the symptoms of their condition. Our study found that nurses were providing guidance to service users on how to adjust their medicines safely in line with how they were feeling:

I have flexibility in how I take my pills. If I feel very sick I stop taking the medicines until I feel better and I always tell the staff what I have been doing. (Male, diagnosed with arthritis)

Case studies

N suffers from diabetes and alters her insulin levels according to her life-style and symptoms. She doesn't like to eat breakfast, and this was difficult to manage with her previous insulin regime. Since seeing the nurse prescriber, she now manages her insulin herself. She consults with the nurse prescriber by phone prior to making any changes to her medication regime.

P alters her medication according to her condition. If she is feeling unwell she 'doubles up' on the dose of her inhaler. If she is suffering with a cold, she takes an extra dose of inhaler in order to 'protect my lungs'.

The ability to self-manage increases feelings of self-efficacy and control and improves quality of life. Nurse prescribers are well placed to promote self-management, ensuring that service users have the flexibility to alter their medicine taking in line with their symptoms, experiences and preferences, without damaging their health or decreasing the effectiveness of their treatment.

Increased access and continuity of care

Ease of access to medication has been found to be a major advantage of nurse prescribing (Luker *et al.*, 1997; Latter *et al.*, 2004). The service users who participated in our study mentioned in particular that they liked having a phone number to contact the nurse if they had side effects from their medicines, new symptoms or general concerns. In their experience, nurses were quite happy to give them a contact number and often suggested it themselves. Even though it was unusual for the nurse to be available to take their call immediately, most had answering machines that they checked regularly, and they would return service users' calls as soon as possible. In a number of cases, service users described ringing their nurse prescriber instead of making an appointment to see a doctor or nurse. They stated that having a nurse prescriber gave then rapid access to advice and information, whereas seeing a doctor always involved booking an appointment through a secretary. Prior to there being nurse prescribers, service users described long waits for appointments and the anxiety this could cause in a crisis.

Some of the service users we interviewed did not have regular access to a medical consultant for specialist advice about their condition, and there were occasions when, even though they had an appointment with a consultant, they actually saw someone else whom they had never met before. For these individuals, the nurse prescriber was their main contact for information about their chronic condition.

There was one particular instance where I discovered some lumps at my insulin injection sites. I immediately rang the nurse prescriber and asked her about them and she reassured me straightaway. Without the nurse I would have panicked. I wouldn't have asked my GP because he doesn't know as much about diabetes as my nurse prescriber does. (Female, diagnosed with diabetes)

We found that service users did indeed view their nurse as the specialist in their care, and this view was shared (and voiced) by both GPs and practice nurses. GPs commonly told service users that nurse prescribers were the 'experts' in their speciality areas and even when patients had contacted their doctor to discuss symptoms or concerns would refer them back to their nurse. For service users requiring frequent adjustments to their medication (for example, those needing insulin), having a nurse prescriber regularly review their medication encouraged adherence to new regimes. Nurse prescribers were considered to have excellent knowledge of the side effects of medicines and of poly-pharmacy issues in their specialty areas.

Reservations about nurse prescribers

Although telephone contact with nurse prescribers increased access to information and advice, service users described difficulties in getting to appointments with their nurse prescribers who were all based in hospitals. They preferred to visit their GP surgery for anything they wanted to discuss in person:

 If I was feeling breathless, I would arrange an appointment with my GP as the first port of call. The GP surgery is more convenient than the hospital as I live close to the surgery. (Female, diagnosed with asthma)

A number of participants in our study were still visiting their GPs to discuss their condition, despite the involvement of a nurse prescriber. This was, in part, due to the proximity of the GP surgery as opposed to the hospital but could also reflect the fact that service users prefer to see a doctor when they are particularly worried about symptoms, or feel that these might indicate a serious problem. It may be that service users view nurse prescribers as the right people to reassure them about minor problems and to answer questions about medication and other treatments but not to deal with serious concerns about their health. Nurse prescribers are valued as a resource for information and advice about chronic health problems, but they must be part of a wider healthcare team that can be easily accessed by the service user. Service users' continued reliance on their GP is illustrated by the story told by one of the participants in our study with a diagnosis of asthma:

The nurse prescriber had recently changed my asthma medication, explaining that I might experience some side effects. However, if I could tolerate the side effects, the medication usually produced good results. I took the new medication as advised but woke up in the night with breathing difficulties. My husband said he had been worried as my breathing seemed to be really shallow. In the morning we immediately made an appointment with my GP to discuss these symptoms. (Female, diagnosed with asthma)

Even though the nurse had explained that there might be some side effects of the new medication, this service user still chose to see her doctor when she became alarmed. Another service user felt quite happy seeing the nurse prescriber for routine care of her chronic health problem but wanted reassurance that the medical consultant was being kept informed about her case and any changes to her care. The desire to see a GP for a 'serious' problem and a nurse for a 'minor' problem has been found in other studies of nurse practitioners/prescribers (Latter *et al.*, 2004; Redsell *et al.*, 2007) and may reflect the fact that service users continue to view nursing as a profession concerned with carrying out delegated tasks and specific procedures.

For the interviewees participating in our study, what mattered was the involvement of the team as a whole in their care, rather than the input of one particular specialist:

Having a nurse prescriber is good as long as she works closely with a specialist and I feel they all know me well. I think I would feel concerned if the nurse prescriber did not have a close relationship with a specialist and she was not able to order and read pathological results. (Female, diagnosed with arthritis)

For the general care of their chronic health conditions, however, most participants described being happy to see the nurse prescriber instead of their doctor:

They do understand, they are knowledgeable and I have no worries that I am receiving a second-class service or being fobbed off. (Male, diagnosed with psoriasis)

They also felt reassured that their nurse would refer them back to the consultant if she had any concerns about their symptoms. The ability of the nurse prescriber to recognise her limitations is important for service users to feel confident in the care that they receive from him or her. The traditional medical hierarchy does not appear to be under any threat with the arrival of nurse prescribing; service users still see doctors as having knowledge superior to that of nurses, even when they describe the nurse as the specialist in their particular condition. Consultants were acknowledged as having extra knowledge in their field, as well as a broad understanding of other conditions, which the nurse prescriber was not considered to possess.

Where a service user has a chronic condition that requires ongoing monitoring and contact with healthcare professionals, they appreciate continuity of the carer. The nurse prescriber was a constant presence in the care of our participants, although they continued to seek out their GPs to supplement their care. Having a nurse prescriber to care for them meant that the interviewees were less reliant on the practice nurses based at the GP surgery. The number of these nurses meant that interviewees were likely to see a different one each time they visited and did not get to know any of them very well. Furthermore, practice nurses were not regarded as having the specialist knowledge of the nurse prescriber; they were considered to be generalists. Practice nurses were also unlikely to be supplementary prescribers and could not make adjustments to medication for service users but had to refer them on to another healthcare professional.

Doctors' perspectives

Although nurses now carry out procedures such as intubation, venesection and minor surgery, which were once the exclusive province of doctors, legislating for them to be able to prescribe has nonetheless generated considerable debate in the UK. In the past, doctors have delegated certain activities to nurses, but non-medical prescribing has been brought in as a government policy, albeit following consultations with medical bodies. The debate, while generally measured, has been illuminating in terms of revealing doctors' perceptions of nurses and other health care professionals [*Pulse* newsletter, 2006). Doctors appear to have strong feelings, both negative and positive, about the appropriateness of nurses becoming prescribers. Some psychiatrists, in common with other specialists, claimed that prescribing for mental health problems was too complex for nurses to undertake and that many of the drug errors reported were due to the administration of medicines by nurses rather than the prescribing of them by doctors (Doran, 2003). The NHS Plan (DoH, 2000) stated the Government's commitment to extend nurse prescribing beyond community and practice nurses. Changes to the Medicines Act were proposed in the Queen's Speech in late 2000, and these paved the way for radical changes to prescribing. In October 2000, the DoH issued a consultation paper on the extension of nurse prescribing, with special mention of mental health (DoH, 2000). The consultation period ended in January 2001, following which the Secretary of State announced that an extra £10 million would be made available to train nurse prescribers between 2001 and 2004.

The Royal College of Psychiatrists' response to the consultation suggested that its members were unhappy about nurse prescribing:

The overwhelming feeling amongst psychiatrists is that psychotropic medication should initially only be prescribed by a psychiatrist acting on their own diagnosis. There may be scope for trained nurses participating in repeat prescriptions and minor modifications thereafter. Prescribing in this area cannot easily be reduced to a few simple rules and there are dangers of omission as well as commission. However, patients should not suffer unnecessarily because of overly rigid rules preventing nurses adjusting medication on the spot. Psychiatrists in Child and Adolescent Psychiatry could not foresee any situation in which it would be appropriate for anyone other than a child psychiatrist to prescribe medication for children and adolescents. In the area of substance misuse, where models of shared care with GPs exist, there may be room for greater flexibility.

Our study sought the views of doctors working in mental health services in the West Midlands 6 years after the Royal College's statement. We conducted a questionnaire survey of all doctors working in three mental health care Trusts. Two hundred and fifty questionnaires were sent out; 149 were returned completed, giving a response rate of 60%. The characteristics of the sample were as follows:

Category	Number	%
Gender		
Male	93	63
Female	54	37
Grade		
Consultant	64	43
Specialist registrars (SpR)	21	14
Middle grade	34	23
Junior doctor	30	20
Age		
23–30	30	20
31–40	47	32
41–50	48	32
50+	24	16

Fifty-eight per cent of doctors who responded felt that nurses should be allowed to prescribe; 27% felt that they should not be allowed to prescribe, and a further 14% were uncertain. For the purposes of analysis, we categorised the doctors as consultants, specialist registrars, middle grade doctors and junior doctors. The questionnaire asked how many years experience respondents had of working in psychiatry; 12% had 1 to 2 years of experience, 16% had 3 to 5 years, 22% had 6 to 10 years, 16% had 11 to 15 years and 34% had more than 5 years of experience. Our analysis of responses indicated that there were a division of opinion between consultants and junior doctors. Seventy-five per cent of consultants agreed that nurses should be able to prescribe, but fewer than 50% of doctors in the lower grades were favourable to the initiative. This cautious attitude may derive from junior doctors being less experienced in the field of mental health and, perhaps, less confident about their future within healthcare teams. Consultants have already gathered a wealth of experience within their specialty, are at the top of their profession and often at the head of their team. Junior doctors, however, have found themselves working in a healthcare system that is constantly changing and 'modernising' and may feel that their position within the system and in their healthcare teams is less secure than was once the case. They now live with the very real possibility that there will be no job for them once they have finished training. The introduction of nurse prescribing challenges the medical status quo and raises the possibility that nurses will take over other aspects of the doctor's role while demanding considerably less pay for doing so. Junior doctors in our study may well have been reflecting anxiously on the attractiveness of non-medical prescribing in a market-driven healthcare economy. As far as the nurse prescribers themselves were concerned, however, their fears were unfounded because the nurses were keen to see themselves as 'maxi-nurses' rather than as 'mini-doctors'.

We asked the doctors to consider whether they felt that nurses should be able to prescribe independently. Whereas 57% of doctors had stated that nurses should be able to prescribe, only 38% agreed that they should be able to prescribe independently. The division between senior and junior doctors was even more apparent in relation to this question, with 54% of consultants, but only 19% of junior doctors, agreeing that nurses should be prescribing independently. We would speculate that these results are further evidence that junior doctors feel threatened by nurse prescribing. There is concern that including nurse prescribers within healthcare teams will reduce the opportunities for junior doctors to gain experience of prescribing, particularly in 'routine' cases for which nurses will increasingly become responsible (Bradley *et al.*, 2007). If junior doctors are unable to gain the experience they need, the problems for the future of medical prescribing are clear.

We probed further into how doctors felt that nurse prescribing could be developed and found more key differences between senior and junior doctors. Forty per cent of junior doctors felt that it would be appropriate to utilise nurse prescribing for out-of-hours care, compared with only 14% of consultants. Over half the junior doctors felt that nurses should be restricted to writing repeat prescriptions, compared with 25% of consultants. Younger doctors (aged 23 to 30 years) were also significantly more likely than older doctors (aged 41 to 50 years) to feel that nurses should be allowed to write only repeat prescriptions. This suggests that younger and more junior doctors are keen to limit nurse prescribing and to keep nurse prescribers under close medical control. Although the younger doctors were more likely than consultants to feel that nurses should be prescribing under medical supervision, this attitude was apparent across the whole group of doctors, two thirds of whom agreed that nurses should be able to prescribe only under medical direction. Nearly a quarter of junior doctors felt that non-medical prescribers should have their practice reviewed on a *daily* basis. This would certainly conflict with the nursing profession's aim to use prescribing as a means of increasing nurses' autonomy in practice and is also at variance with non-medical prescribers' view of their prescribing role as recognition of their expertise in specialist areas such as mental health. There is clearly a possibility that doctors will wish to define the prescribing remit of non-medical prescribers, which could result in non-medical prescribing consisting of large amounts of routine prescribing rather than facilitating responsive, service-user-focussed care. It may be that the desire to monitor nurses' prescribing closely reflects a concern about the assessment and diagnostic skills of non-medical prescribers. By limiting nurses to writing repeat prescriptions in routine cases, doctors would seek to eliminate the need for non-medical prescribers to conduct their own assessments and make diagnoses. Despite this apparent desire to restrict non-medical prescribing, doctors nonetheless acknowledged that nurses had for some time regularly assisted less experienced doctors with prescribing in specialist areas such as mental health. Many would appear to feel more comfortable with nurses remaining in this advisory role rather than becoming prescribers themselves.

When doctors were supportive of non-medical prescribing, key reasons were the potential for decreasing their own workload and for encouraging more effective use of workforce resources across the team. They recognised that non-medical prescribing was acceptable to service users and enhanced their care. However, they were concerned about the training and education of non-medical prescribers, and especially about the generic nature of prescribing courses currently offered in the UK. The courses were described as being too short and failing to provide nurses with the specialist, pharmacological knowledge that doctors felt was necessary to enable them to become safe prescribers. They compared nurses' training with their own and, not unsurprisingly, considered that non-medical prescribing training fell short in terms of the breadth and depth of knowledge provided. There were doubts about the adequacy of nurses' grasp of pharmacology, particularly as the pharmacological content of the nursing pre-registration course has been reduced in favour of more psycho-social models of care. Instead of promoting holistic care, doctors felt that non-medical prescribers could undermine such an approach because they would not have a comprehensive view of treatment options when their knowledge was limited to medicines utilised within their own speciality areas. Because they lacked expertise in other conditions that might affect the service user's presenting, chronic condition, nurses would be unable to take an overview of all symptoms and plan treatment accordingly. Some doctors pointed out that this could be a potentially risky situation because even conditions classified as 'minor' or 'routine' could conceal a more serious diagnosis. To address these potential pitfalls in nurse prescribing, some doctors suggested that nurses should prescribe only within very specific boundaries and using medically negotiated protocols.

There were also concerns expressed by doctors that non-medical prescribing would blur the boundaries between medicine and nursing, leaving room for uncertainty about which professionals should assume overall responsibility for prescribing. This concern may stem from the way in which mental health care was organised historically, with the consultant psychiatrist holding the role of Responsible Medical Officer (RMO) and taking responsibility for the care of all service users. The debate currently taking place about new ways of working includes the suggestion that doctors, whether consultants or GPs, may not always be the most appropriate professionals to take clinical responsibility for every service user (DoH, 2003, 2005). When doctors had overall responsibility for service users, other professionals such as nurses, psychologists and social workers felt that they had little or no influence over the treatments provided and that they occupied a subordinate position in relation to the doctor. Recent policies enable nurses to assume clinical responsibility for some service users, along with rights of admission and discharge. This represents a major attack on the dominance of medical team members not only in mental health care but in other areas of care as well. Prescribing might well be seen by doctors as an additional serious challenge to their authority.

It is not clear from our survey how many of the medical respondents had worked with non-medical prescribers, and this may have shaped their judgement of the prescribing initiative. It is possible that some doctors' opinions will have been informed by the media, discussion in the medical and nursing literature and hearsay. Experience of working alongside someone occupying a new role is a key factor in increasing understanding and acceptance of that role.

Half of the doctors in our survey felt that nurses should be able to prescribe across hospital and community settings. However, two thirds considered it inappropriate to utilise nurse prescribers primarily to provide an out-of-hours service as the nursing literature has suggested might happen in order to compensate for the current shortage of doctors and provide care that doctors do not want to provide. As a result of the general medical services contract (DoH, 2003), many GPs have discontinued their night-time and weekend service, leaving this to be provided by other healthcare workers, including accident and emergency services at local hospitals. If nurses were to take on out-of-hours care, they would certainly need to be able to prescribe, but they would also need a broad range of experience and knowledge. Our survey suggests that doctors feel uncertain that non-medical prescribers have this breadth of practice and are therefore hostile to their providing an out-of-hours service unless heavily supervised and restricted to specific areas.

In considering the potential benefits of nurse prescribing, the responses of the doctors participating in our survey fell into five categories: saving time, enhancing team working, shifting the responsibility for 'routine' care, enhancing patient care and increasing flexibility of response. Doctors supportive of nurse prescribing felt that having a nurse prescriber in their team could free up medical time and prevent duplication of tasks across the team. The potential for non-medical prescribers to take on responsibility for routine cases and repeat prescriptions was seen as an opportunity for doctors to focus their attention on more complex cases. For doctors in favour of non-medical prescribing, nurse prescribing represented a means of introducing new ways of working into their teams; sharing case loads could reduce the overall workload for the team and provide doctors and nurses with a 'second opinion' when needed. With respect to patient care, doctors felt that granting the authority to prescribe to health professionals other than doctors could improve the quality of prescribing care because prescribing decisions would be more widely discussed.

Those doctors who were uncertain about the introduction of non-medical prescribing nonetheless echoed many of the benefits cited by colleagues in favour of the initiative. However, doctors who felt less favourably did not generally consider that a nurse prescriber would give them the opportunity to evaluate how they spent their time, perhaps allowing more time for complex cases and less for routine ones.

The doctors whom we surveyed had mixed views as to whether non-medical prescribing would render care more responsive while maintaining safety standards. Some felt that increased access to medicines might have a negative impact on safety. In a climate where the wishes of service users are paramount, they felt that it was possible that some prescribers might see their role as complying with users' every request, even when what users wanted was not in their best interests. However, many felt that because nurses were effective at communicating with service users about medicines, they had the potential to improve adherence to agreed medication regimens. This benefit would derive from the extra time that doctors felt nurses were able to spend with service users on a one-to-one basis.

Team perspectives

Healthcare services are increasingly provided by teams of healthcare workers whose aim is to work closely together to provide an integrated and effective service responsive to service users' needs. Policy documents such as *New Ways of Working* (DoH, 2005) and *Modernising Nursing careers* (DoH, 2006) have encouraged teams to think about their membership in terms of skills rather than roles and professions. Introducing new roles into teams is a complex process, particularly within a huge organisation such as the NHS. Organisational theorists have found that innovation needs to be undertaken with care and teams kept on board by a constant flow of accurate information; in addition, it is essential that senior management demonstrates its wholehearted commitment to the proposed changes (Edwards, 2000). Non-medical prescribing aims to facilitate greater clinical autonomy within teams and reduce dependence on doctors. However, not all nurse prescribers are working within teams, and some, such as community mental health nurses in rural areas, work in isolation from other team members. Some nurses operate as autonomous practitioners, such as those leading triage services in GP practices. The context of non-medical prescribing is vital to its successful implementation, and access to a supportive team could be crucial in enabling nurses to implement their new role. Within teams, the attitude of team members towards the non-medical prescriber will influence how effectively, or whether, prescribing is utilised in practice. Indeed, supplementary prescribers are unable to prescribe at all unless they have the collaboration of a medical colleague who is prepared to work with them on the CMP.

Team understanding of nurse prescribing

There has been little work conducted with non-medical prescribers to evaluate the impact that team members have on their prescribing practice. We therefore set up focus groups with different teams across the West Midlands.

All the teams invited to participate included a non-medical prescriber (although the prescriber was not invited to the focus group discussion). Teams were drawn from both hospital and community settings and represented five specialty areas – forensic, mental health, learning disability, general practice and neonatal nursing.

All team members exhibited a good understanding of the nurse prescribing role and of how the role was being implemented within their team. Much of this knowledge had been provided by the nurse prescribing team members themselves, and our research certainly suggests that sessions delivered by recently qualified non-medical prescribers to team colleagues to promote their new prescribing roles should be encouraged. Team members particularly appreciated being informed about the remit of individual nurse prescribers' practice because this helped them to consider how best to use her or his skills within the team without stretching them beyond their capacity or expecting them to work outside their scope of practice. Well-informed team members prevented inappropriate referrals being made to the non-medical prescribers and helped teams to explore how best to develop the services they provided.

Despite a good overarching knowledge of non-medical prescribing, team members were confused about the supplementary prescribing role, and particularly the purpose of CMPs. Team members were unclear about the differences between nurses able to prescribe independently and those prescribing only as supplementary prescribers. This confusion is understandable. Although students qualify as both supplementary and independent prescribers, only some will be able to prescribe independently owing to restricted access to the British National Formulary (BNF). Some nurses who could prescribe independently may prefer to work from a CMP while they gain confidence as prescribers. In order to define their prescribing practice clearly, some non-medical prescribers may choose to work from their own 'personal' formulary of medicines. This formulary could be distributed to team members so that they know what the nurse prescriber intends her scope of practice to be, and it could be added to as the nurse prescriber's confidence and experience grow.

Consequences of incorporating nurse prescribing

Aspects of the non-medical prescribing role include reviewing medication regimens, providing expert advice and information about medicines to service users and colleagues, and preventing drug errors and adverse events related to medication. Non-prescribing team members felt that all of these were benefits of having a nurse prescriber in their team and also that an extra prescribing resource saved them and their service users time. This was particularly so for teams in which medical support was scarce and service users would traditionally have to wait a long time for an appointment with a doctor. In GP practices, the nurse prescriber was able to take a lead role in the management of all minor illnesses, usually through offering a triage service, thus freeing doctors to deal with more complex clients.

Nurse prescribers were perceived to be a source of knowledge for the team, and this knowledge sometimes extended beyond issues specific to prescribing. In one learning disability community nursing team, the nurse prescriber had become a source of information about neuropharmacology and polypharmacy but also about the impact that medicine taking could have on the family as a whole. The nurse prescriber in this team was being utilised in a supervisory role to assist less experienced, non-prescribing nursing colleagues. All the teams appreciated that prescribing nurses had a wide range of experience in their specialty areas and increased knowledge about prescribing and medicines. The security that teams gained from the presence of such an experienced person suggests that there should be a commitment to selecting candidates for the prescribing course on the basis of recognised expertise in their areas of practice.

Where non-medical prescribers were working in teams with little medical support, they had become an important resource for the team with respect to prescribing information and medication advice. The non-medical prescribers often knew the service users they were being consulted about and were therefore able to provide advice about medicines grounded in the context of the service user's past experiences and family circumstances. During crises, the non-medical prescriber was perceived as a source of support and advice and was able to initiate treatments in the absence of a doctor. In many instances, the doctors connected to teams changed frequently, and the non-medical prescriber was welcomed for the continuity of support and advice that she or he could provide for the service user and other team members. Team members became familiar with the way that non-medical prescribers thought about medicines and how they made their prescribing choices. As full-time members of the team, they were easily available for consultation with non-prescribing team members in contrast to the sporadic contact that medical prescribers were able to provide.

Having a nurse prescriber in the team was felt to increase debate about medicines across the team as a whole and to improve the safety of prescribing for service users. Such communication was particularly important for teams in which issues to do with polypharmacy were very much to the fore (e.g. in the areas of older adult nursing, learning disability and mental health nursing). One team commented that decision making about medicines had improved since they had gained a nurse prescriber, with colleagues taking more time to think about both pharmacological and non-pharmacological options than they had done previously. There was a feeling that team members were less likely to 'jump to conclusions' and instances were cited of nurse prescribers reducing or stopping drugs without any ill effects on the service user. As a result of this enhanced critique of medicines, teams felt more educated about medicines and that their involvement with prescribing decisions was more considered. All of the non-medical prescribers who participated in our study had selected doctors from within their own teams to be their mentors while training and the benefits of improved liaison and collaborative decision making were felt throughout the team.

The non-medical prescribers were regularly attending seminars and feeding back information to their colleagues. They became an educational resource for their teams, which was particularly valued in the current financial climate of the NHS, which allowed few colleagues the opportunity to attend formal training courses. The potential for the non-medical prescribing role to challenge and redefine other roles within the team was an issue of great interest to the focus groups. One hospital doctor commented that he could see his role evolving into 'medical manager' following the inclusion of non-medical prescribers in teams. The only team that did not provide any examples of team members redefining their roles as a result of non-medical prescribing was the one based in primary care. The nurse prescribing role within this environment was a highly autonomous one, with the nurse leading a triage service and a minor illness clinic. As such, she had less contact on a daily basis with her colleagues.

One of the concerns about extending prescribing rights to healthcare professionals other than doctors has been that prescribing costs will increase. However, the learning disability team who participated in our study felt that they had reduced the level of prescribing since including a non-medical prescriber. The non-medical prescriber did not always prescribe new or additional medicines for service users but saw her role very much as evaluating and reviewing current medication regimens. She worked across the community and spent time in service users' homes looking at the medication that they already had, recommending which should be disposed of, making recommendations about safe storage and ensuring that users' knowledge of their medicines was adequate. She also encouraged her team to give more consideration to non-pharmacological options for treatment. It remains to be seen whether these findings will be replicated in other teams. Prescribing in the area of learning disability is a special case in that there are no specifically designated medicines for the treatment of learning disability and teams rarely have a full-time medical member. However, many service users have co-existing physical conditions such as epilepsy, causing potential problems with polypharmacy. Some service users may have spent years on medicines without ever being reviewed. The potential for non-medical prescribing is considerable in learning disability teams, hopefully encouraging a more holistic approach to client care.

Non-medical prescribers were considered by the participants in the focus groups to have an important role in supporting non-prescribing colleagues. Two of the teams described the nurse prescriber as a key person in promoting team building and improving morale. Team members were inspired to reflect on and develop their own practice because of seeing a nursing colleague successfully complete the prescribing course.

Implementing nurse prescribing within the team

Whether the non-medical prescribing role is successfully implemented in any team depends at least to some extent on the personal characteristics of the prescriber. Nurse prescribers need excellent communication skills to engage service users in discussion about medicines, to explain their role effectively to other team members and to hold their own in discussions with medical team members about prescribing decisions.

Participants in our focus groups recognised that as well as the potential for nurse prescribers to enhance the team's resources, there was also the possibility that they could disable non-prescribing team members. Those non-medical prescribers who had successfully implemented their role had started by sharing caseloads with non-prescribing colleagues rather than taking on their own caseloads for their prescribing practice. This strategy improved service user access to medication whilst also encouraging collaborative working among nursing team members. Focus group participants acknowledged that new prescribers needed time and space to implement prescribing, especially as the seniority of many nurse prescribers ran the risk that their prescribing role would be lost amongst their managerial responsibilities.

Open discussion and debate about advancing nursing roles was felt to be helpful in highlighting concerns about prescribing within the team. Close collaborative working between medical and non-medical prescribers was also seen as important and was assisted by nurses and doctors running clinics together. Objections to nurse prescribing needed to be explored by the team before candidates were sent on the training course.

Team barriers to nurse prescribing

The focus groups, while positive about non-medical prescribing, recognised that it was stretching the boundaries of the traditional nursing role and that some doctors could feel resentful of nurses encroaching on what was traditionally medical territory. Resistance from doctors, although not experienced in any of the teams we spoke to, was felt to be a major barrier to the implementation of nurse prescribing. The full support of all team members and partnership working were thought to be vital to the success of non-medical prescribing.

The number of nurse prescribers within a team has an impact on how effectively the prescribing role is implemented. A single nurse prescriber within a team was unlikely to have a noticeable impact on the service as a whole. Indeed, it was felt that a solitary non-medical prescriber could lead to a two-tier service preventing parity of access to medication for service users. Focus group members suggested the argument that all nurses within a team must be qualified to prescribe, otherwise some users would receive enhanced service while others would have to wait for a medical prescriber to complete their care. Teams in which every nurse could prescribe would find it easier to adopt a consistent approach to the use of medicines, with all team members 'singing from the same hymn sheet' with respect to prescribing practice.

Teams discussed how lack of organisational support, evidenced by the absence of appropriate policies relating to non-medical prescribing, prevented the successful implementation of the role. One team described the difficulty non-medical prescribers were having in accessing computerised prescribing systems. This had led to prescribers choosing not to prescribe independently and reverting to their previous practice of asking a doctor to draw up the prescription for them.

Ongoing education/CPD

Focus group members viewed the non-medical prescriber as accountable and responsible for their practice and therefore obliged to keep up to date with developments in medication. Ongoing education was considered as important for prescribing safety as the training course itself. Meetings with non-medical prescribing peers and mentors, clinical supervision and study days were all suggested as ways in which prescribers could keep themselves well informed. Being able to access information specific to prescribers' specialties was considered to be of key importance. Organisations were felt to be responsible for the provision of this ongoing education and support.

Non-medical prescribers were regarded by focus group members as being proactive in seeking out expert help when they came across a problem. Working in a multi-disciplinary healthcare team enabled them to find many resources for support and information in implementing and extending their prescribing practice. Experienced nurse prescribers were considered to have a vital role to play in supporting newly qualified prescribers.

REFERENCES

Beardon, P. H., McGilchrist, M. M., McKendrick, A. D., McDevitt, D. G. & MacDonald, T. M. (1993) Primary non-compliance with prescribed medication in primary care. *British Medical Journal*, **307**, 846–8.

Billings, A. G. & Moos, R. H. (1981) The role of coping responses and social resources in attenuating the stress of life events. *Journal of Behavioural Medicine*, **4**(2), 139–57.

Bradley, E. J., Pitts, M. K., Calvert, E. & Redman, C. (2001) Illness identity and the self-regulatory model in recovery from early stage gynaecological cancer. *Journal of Health Psychology*, **6**(5), 511–21.

Bradley, E. J. & Nolan, P. (2007) A qualitative study to investigate the impact of nurse prescribing in the UK. *Journal of Advanced Nursing*, **59**(2), 120–7.

Charles-Jones, H., Latimer, J. & May, C. (2003) Transforming general practice: the redistribution of medical work in primary care. *Sociology of Health and Illness*, **25**(1), 71–92.

Department of Health (2000) *The NHS Plan: A Plan for Investment, a Plan for Reform.* London: Department of Health.

Department of Health (2003) *Investing in General Practice: The New General Medical Services Contract.* London: The Stationery Office.

Department of Health (2004) *Management of Medicines: A Resource to Support Implementation of the Wider Aspects of Medicines Management for the National Service Framework for Diabetes, Renal Service and Long-Term Conditions.* July, *http://www.dh.gov.uk/assetRoot/04/08/87/55/04088755.pdf.*

Department of Health (2005) *New Ways of Working for Psychiatrists: Enhancing Effective, Person-Centred Services through New Ways of Working in Multidisciplinary and Multi-Agency Contexts.* London: The Stationery Office.

Department of Health (2006) *Modernising Nursing Careers: Setting the Direction.* London: The Stationery Office.

Doran, C. M. (2003) *Prescribing Mental Health Medication.* London: Routledge.

Edwards, R. (2000) The inevitable future? Post-Fordism in work and learning. In: R. Edwards, S. Sieminski & D. Zeldin (eds), *Adult Learners, Education and Training.* London and New York: The Open University.

Hogg, M. & Vaughan, G. (1995) *Social Psychology: An Introduction.* Melbourne, Australia: Pearson Education.

Johnson, J. (1999) Self-regulation theory and coping with physical illness. *Research in Nursing and Health*, **22**, 435–48.

Latter, S., Maben, J., Myall, M., Courtenay, M., Young, A., Dunn, N. (2004) *An Evaluation of Extended Formulary Independent Nurse Prescribing: Final Report.* Southampton, UK: University of Southampton and Department of Health.

Luker, K. (1997) *Evaluation of Nurse Prescribing. Final Report.* Liverpool: University of Liverpool and University of York.

Miller, A. M. & Mangan, C. (1983) Interacting effects of information and coping style in adapting to gynecologic stress: should the doctor tell all? *Journal of Personality and Social Psychology*, **45**, 223–36.

National Audit Office (2007) *Prescribing Costs in Primary Care.* London: HMSO.

Offredy, M. (2002) Decision-making in primary care: outcomes from a study using patient scenarios. *Journal of Advanced Nursing*, **40**, 532–41.

Pearce, L. (2003) A prescription. *Nursing Standard*, **17**(26), 14–15.

Pulse newsletter 2006. Survey: nurse prescribing a threat to patient safety. *Pulse*, 5 October 2006.

Rashid, A. (1982) Do patients cash prescriptions? *British Medical Journal (Clin Res Ed)*, **284**(6308), 24–6.

Redsell, S., Stokes, T., Jackson, C., Hastings, A. & Baker, R. (2007) Patients' accounts of the differences in nurses' and general practitioners' roles in primary care, **57**, 172–80.

Richman, J. (2002) Keep taking your medication or you will not get better. Who is the non-compliant patient? In: L. Humphries & J. Green (eds), *Nurse Prescribing*, 2nd edn. Basingstoke, UK: Palgrave.

Ridsdale, L., Morgan, M. & Morris, R. (1992) Doctors' interviewing technique and its response to different booking time. *Family Practice*, **9**(1), 57–60.

Venning, P., Durie, A., Roland, M., Roberts, C. & Leese, B. (2000) Randomised controlled trial comparing cost-effectiveness of general practitioners and nurse practitioners in primary care. *British Medical Journal*, **320**, 1048–53.

Vere-Jones, E. (2007) Are patients paying the price? *Nursing Times*, **103**(10), 16–18.

Williams, A. & Jones, M. (2006) Patients' assessments of consulting a nurse practitioner: the time factor. *Journal of Advanced Nursing*, **53**, 188–95.

Pharmacists and prescribing

Amanda Evans

Introduction

This chapter is based largely on the findings from a small-scale study conducted in the West Midlands in early 2005 to explore the experiences and attitudes of seven pharmacist supplementary prescribers (PSPs), their general practitioner (GP) colleagues and practice nurses. All the pharmacists had been qualified as prescribers for a minimum of 6 months at the time of the study and were based in GP practices. Only one of the pharmacists had not yet prescribed. Focus groups and interviews were conducted to explore their readiness to prescribe, their relationships with other practice staff, the feedback they had received from patients, their assessment of their contribution to patient care and any continuing development needs.

The main types of pharmacy practice in the UK comprise community pharmacists ('chemist shop'), hospital pharmacists, pharmacists based in GP practices, Primary Care Trust (PCT)-employed pharmacists (prescribing advisors), industrial pharmacists and academic pharmacists. Practice-based pharmacists (PBPs) are employed to improve the quality and cost-effectiveness of prescribing by offering prescribing advice. In some GP practices, PBPs may also be part of the clinical team and run clinics. Pharmacist supplementary prescribing (PSP) commenced in the UK in 2004, and the sample of PBP prescribers described in this study is made up of the 'pioneers'. As such, the characteristics and practice of these individuals may be different from those of the pharmacy profession as a whole. The early experiences of these pharmacists, and the experiences of colleagues working alongside them, provide essential information about some of the advantages of PSP and barriers to it.

To qualify as a pharmacist, students must complete a 5-year training programme of specialist information in relation to medicines management, pharmaceutics and pharmacology. The standards of education and training for pharmacists are determined and regulated by the Royal Pharmaceutical Society of Great Britain (RPSGB), which has a defined legal and ethical mandate. Pharmacy as a profession experiences the same pressures and incentives to update as other professions within the National Health Service (NHS). The medical profession has historically governed the activities of pharmacists because it is doctors who assess clinical cases and make diagnostic and therapeutic decisions (Denzin & Mettlin, 1968). As a consequence, pharmacists have been slow to establish their unique professional priorities and objectives. Because the requirement for pharmacists to undertake the compounding and small-scale manufacture of drugs has become progressively less important since drug manufacturers started pre-packaging medicines, the pharmacist has, in the opinion of one author, become an 'an over-educated distributor' who merely dispenses prescriptions to patients (Mesler, 1991). Uncertainty about the usefulness of the pharmacist role has led to a situation in which the community pharmacist's work could arguably be accomplished by a qualified technician. Pharmacists are now endeavouring to establish new roles for themselves, such as prescribing, in order to secure their place within the healthcare hierarchy. Because prescribing has previously been one of the core activities of the medical profession (Britten, 2001) and GPs have often relied on prescribing to define their professional effectiveness (Weiss & Fitzpatrick, 1997), it is understandable that some doctors are reluctant for prescribing powers to be 'opened up' to other healthcare groups.

Many pharmacists have sought new positions in different settings away from the traditional chemist shop, becoming prescribing advisors in primary care and prescribers within both primary and secondary care. Such changes have the potential to change the relationship between pharmacist and patient and alter the perceptions of service users. The commercial nature of the local chemist clearly influences how patients perceive pharmacists and the advice that they give about medicines. In a non-commercial environment, such as a GP surgery, pharmacist prescribing advisors may be perceived as more objective. It is likely that pharmacists will have more time to discuss medicines and medicine taking with service users in a clinic setting than they would in a shop, and this will alter the scope of their consultations as well as service user perceptions of their role. These advantages could be viewed as key motivators for pharmacists electing to train as prescribers. Certainly, the maintenance and extension of professions are influenced by professional–public interactions (Friedson, 1972), and prescribing offers an opportunity for pharmacists to redefine and expand their roles.

Pharmacists themselves have key attributes that fit them well for the role of prescriber. Their training means that they have good pharmacological knowledge. Pharmacist prescribers in primary care commonly hold postgraduate clinical qualifications in addition to their prescribing qualification and pharmacy degrees. This represents a huge amount of time spent studying pharmacology in comparison to the time allocated to this subject in the training of doctors and nurses. Pharmacists must adhere to protocols and ethical boundaries and are required to be systematic. These are skills and attributes of immediate relevance to supplementary prescribing when the care management plan (CMP) must be written and delivered in a systematic manner.

In their traditional role of supplying medicines to service users, pharmacists were already using key skills related to prescribing, such as discussing scripts with service users to highlight potential co-morbidities and drug interactions and applying prescribing evidence before allowing scripts to be dispensed.

Pharmacist prescribers generally assert that they do not want responsibility for making diagnoses, and they have shown little interest in taking further training to enable them to become diagnosticians. Now that pharmacist prescribers are able to qualify as *independent* prescribers, it will be interesting to see whether they change their position on diagnosis.

The pioneers

In the UK, most pharmacists who have presented for prescribing training have come from hospital or primary care backgrounds (including GP practice–based pharmacists and those employed by PCTs); fewer community pharmacists have sought prescribing training. This is somewhat ironic, given that most healthcare provision is now located in community settings. It may be that the smaller number of community pharmacists seeking training relates to a shortage of medical practitioners providing clinical mentorship for this group. PSPs must spend around 90 hours of their training working closely with a doctor in a clinical prescribing setting. However, there is currently no funding available for doctors to undertake these roles. In addition, few community pharmacists work closely with doctors, compared with hospital or practice-based pharmacists, and they may therefore experience difficulty finding doctors willing to support them during their training. Finally, community pharmacists are not required to top up their education with a clinical pharmacology diploma, whereas many hospital and practice-based pharmacists already hold this postgraduate qualification and may therefore feel less daunted by the additional therapeutic and pharmacological knowledge required to undertake prescribing. There is little evidence to suggest how much and what type of work would be available to pharmacists prescribing within chemist shops; therefore, community pharmacists may perhaps be inclined to wait for pioneers to clarify the role before applying to train themselves (Andalo, 2003).

A large, national study conducted by George *et al.* (2006) involved a self-completed questionnaire sent to all newly qualified pharmacist prescribers on the RPSGB's register. There were 518 responses. The results showed that prescribing pharmacists were mostly female (67.3%), 30.7% had more than 20 years of experience, 40% worked in hospital settings and over a third (35.7%) specialised in cardiovascular conditions. Nearly half had prescribed in practice, with over half (58.4%) of the prescriptions being written in primary care settings. These findings resemble those relating to nurse prescribers, who have been predominantly women with many years in practice. Nurses working in primary care settings produce far more prescriptions than those working in other environments.

The seven pharmacist prescribers who participated in this study had all elected voluntarily to undertake the training course and were happy to be regarded as prescribing 'pioneers'. Six were self-funding and were prepared to implement prescribing practice in the absence of any guiding models. All participant prescribers stated that they wanted to become prescribers because this would give them greater satisfaction in the work they were doing. For example, one of the participants had been running a multi-disciplinary hypertension clinic for 5 years. Post-qualification, the pharmacist was able to manage all aspects of the clinic, including prescribing, and provide a total care package to service users. Since the advent of independent pharmacist prescribing in 2007, some of the original population of supplementary prescribers have gone on to qualify as independent prescribers, but only as an adjunct to their original practice-based pharmacist role.

It was uncommon for the PSPs in our study to be employed solely as 'prescribers'; they were more likely to have 'portfolio' careers with a range of roles to fulfil, only one of which was prescribing. This situation is similar to that of nurse prescribers in both primary and secondary care, whose prescribing practice is defined by the environment within which they work and complements other roles rather than taking over as a primary role. It is unlikely that full-time pharmacist prescribing roles will be commissioned until pharmacist prescribing has been more fully 'rolled out' and evaluated across the UK. The cost-effectiveness of pharmacist prescribing will be a primary factor in the creation of such roles and of particular concern to commissioners.

Participants in focus groups conducted to explore the impact of prescribing in practice found that PSPs experienced various challenges in implementing their new role. They did not feel that being prescribers generated respect from peers or other professional colleagues, and they felt heavily dependent on existing personal contacts with colleagues for support. This situation would present difficulties for PSPs who have changed their jobs or moved into new teams in order to become prescribers, who do not have supportive team members around them. Until there is a larger 'critical mass' of PSPs, organisations must consider the types of support new PSPs require and how to provide it in practice.

Pharmacists working in hospitals before commencing their prescribing training reported that they had already been engaged in 'virtual prescribing'; they were used to making prescribing decisions and then waiting for a doctor to write out the prescription. These pharmacists felt that acquiring the PSP qualification was essentially a "rubber stamp" exercise to legitimise their existing practice.

However, a huge difference was found between what primary care pharmacists in training hoped to be doing once qualified and what they found themselves doing on completion of the course. That was largely due to the way in which primary care pharmacists have traditionally been employed by primary care organisations and GPs, namely, to ensure cost-effective prescribing rather than provide services directly to patients. No matter how much pharmacist prescribers may have aspirations to work as diabetic specialists, for instance, this role is generally not open to them unless they can demonstrate that they can implement it in such a way as to achieve savings for the employing organisation.

So strong is this directive to be of financial assistance to the organisation that PSPs tend to see themselves as assistants to doctors, defining their activities in terms of how useful they are to doctors rather than in terms of their contribution to the service overall. While PSPs are pleased to have the opportunity to enjoy a more inclusive relationship with other healthcare professions, they still feel that they are "outsiders". To date, few report that they are fully integrated into healthcare teams in primary care settings. Those who have become fully integrated have done so by virtue of their own efforts in forging professional relationships and demonstrating to colleagues the 'added value' they can bring to decision making and overall quality of care delivered.

What motivated pharmacists to become prescribers?

Key attributes
Given their level of training and the nature of the work they do, it is not surprising that many PSPs claim that they have greater knowledge of medication management than GPs or nurses. Some see their role primarily as educational, advising doctors and nurses about drugs, especially in instances when patients may have more than one problem. Many perceive that they are experts in identifying appropriate drugs for specific conditions, recognising drug reactions, predicting and recognising the interactions of several drugs, and recommending ways in which drug treatment can be optimised. They are confident about making decisions on complex drug-related therapies involving more than one area of medicine, such as identifying and managing a medicines regimen for a pregnant woman who also has a cardiovascular problem and schizophrenia. These skills enable 'complex problems' to be dealt with, with a degree of sophistication not always evident in the past when such patients were seen by different specialists, each having little knowledge of what other specialists were prescribing.

Different relationship with patients
PSPs felt that they relate to patients very differently from the way in which other professional colleagues relate to them. Their focus is on the medicines being prescribed and on the understanding that patients have about what is being

prescribed for them. They try to start from where patients are at in terms of their understanding of their condition, what treatments they expect to be prescribed and what they believe the purpose of treatment is. Pharmacists contend that they involve the patient more in decisions about choice of medicine than doctors do because they are aware of a variety of pharmacological ways of treating different conditions, depending on the person's lifestyle. Pharmacists increase patients' knowledge of their medicines and hence extend the choices they can make. This approach results in greater concordance of patients with medication regimens than is achieved by other professionals. PSPs consider that while they may be perceived as expensive in the short term, owing to the amount of time they devote to each patient, in the long term they are cost-effective because of the levels of concordance achieved, better long-term management of chronic conditions and their capacity to motivate people to take an interest in the management of their health. All seven respondents affirmed that when prescribing decisions are negotiated, health outcomes are better.

The PSPs who participated in this study reported that patients discussed their feelings about their medicines with them with more honesty and questioning than they had when they were practice-based pharmacists. Prescribing meant seeing patients more often and having a 'different, and better, relationship' with them. Prior to becoming prescribers, they would see a patient at most once a year; now they were seeing them at least once a month and so could negotiate a deeper relationship with patients, even those who were initially hesitant about seeing a pharmacist prescriber. Commenting on this, one PSP said:

After a couple of visits, they're very, very happy and they want to stick with it quite often. I mean the difficulty now is actually discharging people.

Many of the PSPs indicated how dissatisfied they had been with their previous roles, which required them to advise doctors and nurses about how to derive maximum benefits from drug treatments but did not allow them to make these changes directly. As prescribers, they felt they were more engaged in a *process* of caring for patients, which resulted in their feeling more satisfied because they could see the impact of treatment:

As a supplementary prescriber...the decision now is a negotiation between myself and the patient, without any interference from anybody else. A patient might say,..."I don't like the taste of that tablet that you're suggesting'...That could possibly floor me as a practice pharmacist because plan A has gone...but I've got the authority as a supplementary prescriber to actually find a way through this minefield – with the patient's help. That makes a big difference to me.

Because pharmacists are now in a position to make their own decisions about patients' medication, they enjoy more clinical autonomy than previously, although still limited by the CMP. Being able to make changes to a patient's med-ication without having to consult others is a considerable step and something about which the PSPs felt very positively. Some now want full clinical autonomy and are training to become independent prescribers. While they can see merits in having a CMP, they find it a barrier to taking their new relationship with patients to the next level.

Key benefits of becoming a prescriber

The PSPs themselves felt that their greatest strength as prescribers was the pharmacological knowledge they brought to the management of patients with chronic conditions and to those requiring complex medication regimens. This breadth and depth of pharmacological knowledge enabled them to advise the team on combinations of medicines, the frequency with which blood levels needed to be checked, the advice that patients should receive and how often patients should be seen for follow-up. Many of the PSPs considered that their time was deployed to best effect in supporting others and attending meetings where decisions were made about complex treatment plans.

In addition to giving advice, PSPs in this study either worked in or ran a variety of clinics:

- Hypertension – for patients not responding to standard treatments or who had complex co-morbidities or needs
- Anti-coagulation
- Dyspepsia (these clinics were popular with PCTs because of the huge cost savings they allow)
- Medication review
- Substance misuse
- Coronary heart disease, usually involving more complex cases
- Smoking cessation, largely because 'no one else wanted to do it'.

Having higher status

All the respondents believed that undertaking additional training and radically altering the focus of their practice meant that the status of their work had increased. This brought the issue of remuneration into consideration:

if you think we're doing part of the doctor's job in some way. . . . I think really we should actually be paid a higher rate, but we're not.

Pharmacists, in contrast to nurses, continually define their new role *in relation to that of doctors*, and this re-evaluation inevitably highlights the fact that doctors are paid considerably more than pharmacists. Being able to work directly with patients and intervene as appropriate with their treatment has had the effect of reinvigorating the pharmacists' role and expanding it into what was previously the domain of doctors.

Greater job satisfaction

Considering where their new role might take them in the future, the PSPs were unanimous in agreeing that their job satisfaction had increased. This is a function both of working as part of the healthcare team and of having more control over what they do. Receiving recognition from other healthcare professionals and from patients is gratifying. Interestingly, the PSPs noted that what others found most helpful was the pharmacological knowledge they had acquired during undergraduate and postgraduate training rather than their ability to prescribe. This confirms what many pharmacists have felt for some time, namely, that they are, and have been for decades, an under-used resource in the NHS:

I think over the years that pharmacist skills have not been totally utilised and supplementary prescribing is a way forward, for us to come out, you know, to prove what we can do and contribute to the healthcare team.

It seems logical that at a time when drugs are increasingly central to treatment, there should be at least one member of the clinical team with specific expertise in medication.

Being part of the primary healthcare team

Many practice pharmacists work sessionally and are not directly employed by the practice in which they work. Traditionally, the PCT has employed them, determining the nature and scope of work they undertake. Being employed by one organisation and working in another can be a source of frustration and disagreement. Some of the PSPs who took part in this study, however, were practice employees and worked to the agenda set by the GPs. They took pleasure in being part of the team and enjoyed feeling less on the periphery of the NHS. One respondent noted a raft of benefits arising from this:

Since being part of the team, I am now invited to the Christmas Party, team outings and staff meetings. For the first time in my life, I have my own room, my own computer and whatever equipment I need. I also can use the 'appointments system' to arrange when I need to see patients. By virtue of what I have been given and what I do, I feel I am a valued member of the team and my status has increased enormously.

Feeling a member of the team, in the way described above, is dependent on the existing team accommodating the pharmacist and creating the conditions in which he or she feels included. When teams are welcoming, pharmacists wish to make as significant a contribution as possible. As for nurse prescribers, the environment in which the pharmacists work when assuming their new prescribing role is of the utmost importance.

A GP who contributed to the study described how their pharmacist was accepted as a supplementary prescriber 'more by default' than as a result of the practice's strategy:

The practice pharmacist, having completed the course, canvassed, really, to see if he could do some chronic disease management.

All the PSPs had made direct approaches to the practices in which they now worked. None had been approached by the practices. This had been a necessary strategy to adopt in locating their first appointment as prescribing pharmacists.

Putting prescribing into practice

All the PSPs who participated in the study agreed that, on becoming part of the team, they had to adopt the system of working that was already in place. This meant conforming to the times decided by the practice for when they should conduct their clinic work. The appointment system took into account when people were available, the availability of rooms and when patients were able to attend. While there were adequate resources for the team, this did not mean that resources were always available for individuals.

Invited to comment on their first experiences of prescribing, the PSPs identified the following areas as important.

Accommodation
Each PSP was allocated a consulting room in which to see patients. Whereas doctors tended to keep the same room, other professionals were more likely to share or simply to be allocated a room that was free on a given day. Room sharing or 'desk hopping' was a feature of many of the primary care services discussed by the PSPs because there were always more personnel than rooms. They had full co-terminal access to patient records and some had access to diagnostic equipment, although four had to purchase their own.

Information technology (IT) support
In general, IT support was considered to be poor. Five of the PSPs had to handwrite prescriptions and then annotate patients' records. This was found to be an unsatisfactory and time-consuming practice. Some had to buy their own equipment, which did not assist their integration with other members of the practice.

Hours
None of the PSPs worked full time as prescribers; all had other jobs to do. Four worked 2 days a week in primary care, and two worked 2.5 days. One was also a community (chemist shop) pharmacist and worked half a day as a PSP.

Types of patients seen
The PSPs took on the management of particular patients, prescribing for them for a pre-determined time period only. Some took on patients for about 3 months

until they were stabilised – for example, managing patients on antihypertensive medication until their blood pressure was under control. Others were able to prescribe for up to a year.

Patient referrals

The process by which PSPs were allocated patients varied considerably. Some were allocated 2 or 3 patients at a time, while others had up to 30; some PSPs waited for patients to be allocated to them, others identified the patients that they wished to see. When this happened, the PSPs were expected to ask the GP's permission to take on the role of prescriber for those particular patients. In practices where there were multiple partners, it was usual for two or three GP 'champions' to willingly refer patients to the pharmacists. GPs who were reluctant to refer tended to wait and see how the PSPs conducted their work before referring patients to them. Once a PSP had demonstrated that she or he was competent and appreciated by patients, the more cautious GPs were then making referrals. During the period of this study, no nurses referred to pharmacists, and neither did all GPs in every practice.

Workload

When the practice was paying for the services of pharmacist, it determined the work the pharmacists would do. Other PSPs reported that it was left to them to manage their time and choose what they wanted to be involved with. They did not experience any interference from GPs. However, all the GP employers expressed concern to the PSPs about getting value for money in terms of benefit to patients.

Reimbursement

A range of financial models was deployed by practices to remunerate the pharmacists. These included being paid directly by the GP practice and being paid by the PCT. Some stated that they were self-employed and did "sessional work" when they were able to. Another stated that he had a short-term contract, and one said he was on secondment from the PCT to the GP surgery. Although these variations did not apparently cause any concerns to the pharmacists, they may affect the extent to which they see themselves as part of a team.

Prescribing, not diagnosing

The PSPs readily acknowledged that, especially in complex conditions, diagnosing could be difficult and often required specialised investigations and assessments. They recognised that they did not have the same level of diagnostic skills as doctors but felt this was not a barrier to their becoming prescribers. Whereas doctors tend to see prescribing as inextricably linked to diagnosis, PSPs do not agree with their argument that to separate diagnosis from prescribing is illogical.

Those who participated in the study were content that diagnosis should remain the prerogative of doctors.

Pharmacist prescribers – a different style of patient management

A national study of prescribing pharmacists conducted by George *et al.* (2006) found that 71.3% of the sample claimed that improved patient management was the main contribution to be made by PSPs. The PSPs in our study also considered that they, compared with doctors, were better at negotiating treatments with patients. In studies carried out by Lundkvist *et al.* (2002) around the subject of communication between patients and healthcare professionals, it was found that although doctors did initiate discussions about treatment with their patients, they tended to dominate the discussion. They did not always name the drug they were prescribing or explain how new drugs differed in mechanism or purpose from those previously prescribed. They did not usually check patients' understanding of treatments or explore their concerns. When they did encourage patients to ask questions, the patients seldom did so. Doctors discussed the benefits of treatment more than the risks or precautions needing to be taken or patients' ability to follow the treatment plan. The study reported that patients were not given sufficient information about the medicines they were taking, and those who asked were often dissatisfied with what they were told.

The PSPs interviewed for the study described here were of much the same opinion. They felt that they involved the patient more than doctors in decisions about the choice of medicine and were as keen to help patients understand both their treatment and their condition. This may be because the PSPs usually offered longer consultation times than did doctors (20 minutes compared with less than 10). Like nurse prescribers, the PSPs believed that longer consultations meant that they were able to have a more in-depth conversation with their patients about treatment, and this in turn affected the quality of current and aftercare that patients received.

Concordance centres on patients being sufficiently informed so that they can make appropriate decisions about their health and treatment. Paternalism, characteristic of old-fashioned medicine, does not allow patient-centred care and is being replaced by an approach which seeks to educate, involve and empower patients so that they have an investment in their own recovery. Martin *et al.* (1999) and Freeman *et al.* (2002) confirmed that the longer the consultation time (20 minutes and over), the more dialogue was initiated by patients. Dialogue concerned how to live with an illness and how to get the best treatment from taking certain medicines. Longer consultations are particularly important for patients with complex and/or chronic conditions who need time to review their illness and treatment as well as the opportunity to discuss how their personal management strategies could be improved. The PSPs interviewed in this study considered that they were better than doctors at negotiating medication regimes because there was less social distance between patients and pharmacists, so patients were able to be honest about treatment lapses rather than deferential.

Barriers to pharmacists becoming prescribers

In autumn 2005, there were around 500 qualified pharmacist supplementary prescribers (DoH, 2005). Slightly fewer than half were actually prescribing, the chief obstacle being funding, which was identified by 71 of the pharmacists (36.4%) in the study of prescribing pharmacists made by George *et al.* (2006). The second most common barrier was reported to be organisational problems, as identified by 37 (18%). Other factors that presented barriers included frustration at not being able to commence prescribing as soon as the pharmacists had finished training, lack of confidence in their ability to prescribe, working in an alien environment and working with patients whom they had little experience of treating. This study left no doubt that merely attending a prescribing course does not prepare pharmacists for working in clinical practice, and much support was required if they were to implement their prescribing qualification. Hospital pharmacists were far more likely to be practising as PSPs a year after training than those working in community settings. This may have been because they were well supported by colleagues and clinical mentors with whom they had already formed close working relationships. Many of the same issues were highlighted by the study described in this chapter.

Funding issues

The primary concern for the PSPs was the absence of specific prescribing budgets for pharmacists, meaning that they were obliged to prescribe from medical budgets. Under the terms of the General Medical Services contract, many GPs are at a loss to understand how employing a prescribing pharmacist can be cost-effective. There is no additional funding for growth or innovation because there is under the Personal Medical Services contract. Nurse prescribers, who can be employed at band 5, are far less expensive than pharmacist prescribers, who generally start at band 7. So unless pharmacists can put forward a convincing business case, demonstrating the financial benefits of their employment, they are unlikely to be taken on. Many pharmacist prescribers have managed to do this; they *have* demonstrated that they can provide services that are both clinically effective and cost-effective in primary care settings. However, three of the participants in this study commented that the doctors they had approached remained unconvinced. The pharmacists were also deeply concerned about the lack of funding for clinical mentors. Pharmacists who would like to undertake prescribing training cannot do so because they are unable to find a doctor willing to give them clinical mentorship without being reimbursed for the considerable commitment in time this represents.

Lack of support

The PSPs expressed anxiety about how they were perceived by other team members. They felt that pharmacy practice within primary care was seen as marginal and not central to the work of the healthcare team. Even practice-based prescribing pharmacists, who have strong links with other team members, considered that they were valued primarily because of the cost savings they could bring about and not because they were seen as clinical equals. Their clinical involvement often took the form of medication reviews, or one-off encounters with patients. If they had no real opportunity to forge relationships with the patients attending the practice, their job satisfaction could be poor. It is a major challenge for pharmacists to be accepted as full members of the clinical team.

Many of this first generation of pharmacist prescribers had found their own route to gaining employment as prescribers. Some had argued with their employing organisations that by allowing them to write prescriptions, they could improve patient access to medicines and achieve savings of time and costs. Others had used existing relationships with GPs to be allowed to "dabble" in prescribing. A few had tried to convince their PCTs to give them a "trial" period as prescribers. However, *none* of the PSPs had been encouraged to become prescribers by either their employing organisations or their non-pharmacist colleagues. All were self-motivated, and most had funded their training themselves.

At the time of undertaking this study, there were no DoH directives about the benefits of employing PSPs. Neither commissioners nor PCTs were taking any interest in prescribing pharmacists and most pharmacists themselves lacked interest in the prescribing initiative. No PCTs had considered the possibility of devising competency assessments to show what the health gains for patients and carers might be if prescribing pharmacists were employed. Those PSPs participating in the study who *had* found employment as prescribers stated that they had received little or no support from their employers in terms of clinical governance, risk analysis, support following significant events, access to steering groups or access to peer support groups. Very few had operational guidelines from either their PCT or their employers:

It feels as though we are ploughing a furrow through very deep snow.

Few prescribing pharmacists were being invited to take part in critical event meetings at their practices. With no opportunities to report, comment, reflect on and learn from critical incidents and the outcome of risk assessments, the pharmacists admitted to feeling very vulnerable. This was cited as the main reason for withdrawing from running special clinics. The lack of prescriber forums and ongoing clinical mentorship was keenly felt.

Technical/operational difficulties

Newly qualified PSPs described their frustration at not being able to gain full access to the clinical systems at the GP surgeries, or even to patients' notes. Some prescribing pharmacists had to use the name of colleague to gain access to the system. Another irritation was the time it took for them to be issued with a prescription pad. When the pads finally arrived, they were pre-printed by the prescribing authorities and could not be run through the clinical system's printer. This meant that the patients' drugs had to be hand copied onto the pads from the printed screen, running the risk of transcription errors as well as being time-consuming.

Despite pressure from government to increase the number of pharmacist prescribers, the first prescribers had great problems in obtaining appropriate professional indemnity insurance. When the indemnity finally became available, some self-funding pharmacists found cost prohibitive and discontinued their prescribing practice.

Doubts about the usefulness of pharmacist prescribing

In the letters pages of the pharmaceutical press, many pharmacists argued that to become prescribers would entail a considerable investment of time with no certain benefits in view (Axon, 2003). This discussion generated a wait-and-see attitude in many pharmacists. Their doubts were further fuelled by the medical profession, which questioned whether it was appropriate for pharmacists to be prescribing at all. They suggested that pharmacists lacked both diagnostic skills and what were regarded as the more fundamental skills of 'relating to' and 'knowing' the patient. How pharmacists 'see' patients and how they 'get to know' them has received relatively little attention to date. It is now imperative that pharmacist prescribers address the 'patient factor' before inter-professional doubts about their prescribing abilities can be overcome (Buckley *et al.*, 2006).

The views of the medical profession

The interviews with participants in this study leave little doubt that entry for non-medical personnel into prescribing practice in primary and secondary care in the UK is controlled by doctors. Some doctors do not feel that pharmacists are the most appropriate healthcare professionals to prescribe. This would appear, at least in part, to be related to misunderstanding of the roles of pharmacists. Ignorance of what other professionals do is prevalent in healthcare. Lloyd *et al.* (2005) found that more than two thirds of hospital doctors were unaware of the role of a supplementary prescriber. The British Medical Association (BMA, 2005) 'reacted with dismay' when independent prescribing by nurses and pharmacists was announced, labelling this development as highly irresponsible on the part of government and potentially dangerous for patients (Avery & Pringle, 2005).

As part of this study, 10 GPs were interviewed about PSPs; 7 felt positively but 3 expressed grave reservations about the role of pharmacists as prescribers.

The main points to emerge from three focus groups with GPs were that:

- GPs were uncertain about relinquishing control of prescribing.
- They were happy to delegate certain aspects of patient care to pharmacists as long as they retained overall control of the care of patients.
- One group felt that if they allowed pharmacists to prescribe, practices would be more vulnerable to clinical risks.
- Some were concerned that pharmacists might not see enough patients to make their clinics pay.
- Diagnosis is a key element of the prescribing process, and pharmacists do not posses diagnostic skills. The training course is for prescribing, not diagnosing.
- One group of GPs expressed doubts about the selection process. They did not like the idea of pharmacists self-selecting for the prescribing course.
- GPs did not want community pharmacists to be prescribers because they felt that the chemist shop was an inappropriate setting for prescribing.
- Some GPs were concerned about the speed of implementation of non-medical prescribing, describing it as 'scary'.
- Many GPs said that they would rather employ a nurse prescriber than a pharmacist prescriber.

Hughes and McCann (2003) identified that some GPs see the pharmacist as merely a 'shopkeeper' and believe that the commercial imperative of the chemist shop prevents honest clinical interventions. The finding that GPs have doubts about the skills of pharmacists and a lack of awareness of the extent of training they have undertaken was echoed in the study reported in this chapter. Like the study of Hughes and McCann, the present study also found that GPs trust practice pharmacists more because of the absence of commercialism in their interactions with patients.

PSP has been a government-driven initiative, with the backing of the RPSGB. Some GPs have perceived a hidden agenda to undermine the medical profession's power so that clinical decisions are increasingly determined by bureaucratic control. Medicine can be subject to rationalisation, which is where it is broken down into separate, technical tasks, one of which is prescribing, which can be taken away from doctors and performed by less highly paid professional groups such as pharmacists (McKinlay, 1977). Pharmacist prescribing is also seen by some as one of many Government interventions of the last two decades which some doctors view as threats to their professional and clinical autonomy. Professional autonomy has been defined as the legitimated control that an occupation exercises over the organisation and terms of its work (Elston, 1991).

Other examples of outside intervention are the fundholding/indicative pre-scribing budgets later superceded by PCT prescribing budgets managed by pre-scribing advisers. Under this system, PCT local formularies and clinical gover-nance are maintained by medical peers at PCT level (or by PCT pharmacists) and are used to challenge expensive or poor prescribing practice. More recently the new General Medical Services contract contains a quality outcome framework based on a point scoring system which directs practice activity at specific ther-apeutic and clinical targets. This is a further challenge to the clinical autonomy of the doctors.

In the face of these changes, it is understandable that non-medical prescribing may be seen by GPs as a further challenge to traditional medical hegemony and the doctors' dominance over allied healthcare professions. There has been a gradual encroachment on doctors' prescribing activities since what has been termed, 'the heydays of the 1970s'. Some physicians view further changes in the traditional relationship between pharmacists and doctors with alarm.

There are precedents to this type of 'boundary encroachment' (a term coined by Eaton and Webb in 1979) by pharmacists on the doctors' territory. During the seventies, clinical pharmacists in hospitals attempted to extend the boundaries of pharmacy into the territory of doctors, capitalizing on their pharmacological knowledge and providing advice and information about medicines to patients, doctors and nurses. This involved face-to-face contact with patients on all mat-ters concerned with their medication, and 'enhancing the ability of physicians to make good decisions about medicines'. At first there were some occupational difficulties for these early clinical pharmacists in their relationships with the medical profession, but the medical profession negotiated a settlement in rela-tion to this initiative in its favour by controlling the activities of the pharmacists as a form of delegation (Turner, 1987). By the early 1990s, the clinical phar-macists working in hospitals had been largely accepted, and both doctors and nurses had come to welcome the expertise in medication therapy that hospital pharmacists could provide.

Friedson (1972) has noted a potential conflict between physicians and phar-macists in modern times. Pharmacy is a profession which provides services related to healing; if unregulated or deregulated, it might, as in earlier centuries, find itself in competition with the practice of physicians. He suggests that the services of pharmacists are necessary to the practice of physicians and poten-tially a threat to their position. The medical profession is therefore driven to ensure that pharmacists' activities are circumscribed in order to maintain the dominance of doctors.

Eaton and Webb (1979) further suggested that, historically, the medical pro-fession has maintained its supremacy over related professions by systematic expansionism and delegation. It expands to incorporate new disciplines in order to retain dominance over those disciplines' practitioners. This pattern of behaviour can be seen in relation to nurse prescribers; doctors have welcomed them – provided that they remain under the control of their employing GP practices. If this theory is held to be correct, it is not surprising that PSP, and more recently independent prescribing, are viewed with distrust by some sections of the medical community.

The evidence from the GP focus groups in this study suggests that GPs feel relatively comfortable with nurse extended roles in their practices. Although there was some ambivalence about nurse prescribing, there was far more about pharmacist prescribing. This may result from the fact that nurse prescribing is more readily accepted by GPs because of the relationship and boundaries that exist between themselves and practice nurses. Because doctors and nurses have traditionally shared some of their trainings both in hospital and practice settings, there is a high level of understanding of each other's roles. Pharmacists' training, on the other hand, is far less visible to doctors, and it may be difficult for GPs to identify a role for prescribing pharmacists because so many practices already employ prescribing nurses. The pharmacists who have been successful in primary care settings have tended to identify something that neither doctors nor nurses want to do, such as treating pharmacologically challenging patients who have complicated and/or chronic diseases.

Factors that enable pharmacists to take up prescribing in primary care

Despite a lot of negative press in the medical literature, there are GPs who are able to see the opportunities inherent in pharmacist prescribing. Once funding issues are resolved (and practice-based commissioning may be the way forward for pharmacists) and models of pharmacist prescribing practice are established, more GP practices are likely to wish to employ a pharmacist prescriber and provide mentorship to prescribing students. The picture portrayed in this chapter is one which existed at the very beginning of pharmacist supplementary prescribing in one part of the country, and it is possible that, were the same study to be undertaken now, a different picture might emerge. GPs will be influenced by the apparent popularity of pharmacist prescribing with patients. Chen and Britten (2000) found that patients are eager to discuss their medication in detail with pharmacists, as emerged from the study reported here. As an increasing number of pharmacists demonstrate that successful prescribing partnerships can be established in primary care, other pharmacists will be encouraged to present themselves for prescribing training and GPs will become more interested in employing PSPs. Primary care Trusts, where there is an influential pharmaceutical advisor or pharmacist, may take a lead in setting up pilot sites for PSP clinics. These will give PSPs the opportunity to demonstrate their usefulness without any financial risk to the practices within which they are based.

Four years since the arrival of pharmacist supplementary prescribing, there is better support from the pharmaceutical organisations for prescribing pharmacists. Online prescriber forums are established; template business plans for would-be PSP clinics are available; there is a competency framework for PSP, published by the National Prescribing Centre, which identifies pharmacists' training needs, and most importantly, there is a clinical governance framework from the RPSGB, which was published in 2006. More PCTs are being supportive in terms of providing operational guidelines, steering groups and peer support groups for PSPs.

The future of pharmacist prescribing

Independent prescribing became legal on 1 May 2006, with pharmacists in England being allowed to prescribe any licensed medicine (except controlled drugs) without clinical management plans. With these new arrangements, some might ask whether there is any ongoing need to take supplementary prescribing into account. This question was tackled by Matt Griffiths, joint Prescribing Adviser at the Royal College of Nursing, at a conference on non-medical prescribing in London in May 2006. Griffiths predicted that supplementary prescribing will remain useful for patients with complicated conditions. It may be a means of newly qualified prescribers gaining competence and confidence and of training staff in how to prescribe for new conditions. It is believed that supplementary prescribing will increase adherence because patients will be more involved in their own care.

Currently, a major obstacle preventing pharmacist prescribing from being more widely accepted is the lack of evidence of the added value that it brings to clinical practice. The RPSGB needs to consider creating an evidence-based model to enhance the professional standing of pharmacist prescribing. This, in turn, will assist the employment opportunities for pharmacist prescribers within a context of practice-based commissioning.

Granby (2003) has observed that pharmacist prescribers must have the opportunity to prescribe on a regular basis so that they develop and maintain the competency and confidence needed to prescribe safely and effectively. There are gaps in provision in primary care that pharmacists could fill, for example, by providing out-of-hours service. Patients often put pressure on community pharmacists to supply prescription drugs without a prescription during out-of-hours periods. One solution is for pharmacists to be allowed to prescribe within pre-agreed protocols.

Pharmacist prescribing, in line with all non-doctor prescribing, would benefit from greater support. PCTs must ensure that clinical governance and competency frameworks are in place and establish operational support systems that include mentoring, peer groups and prescribing forums. The findings from the study reported here make it clear that non-medical prescribers need access to patients' records. This was a hot topic in the Drugs and Therapeutics Bulletin throughout 2006 because electronic medical records are not expected to be fully rolled out in England until 2010.

Better collaboration between non-medical prescribers would strengthen all parties. Such links can be created by setting up multi-disciplinary clinics, a few of which are already in existence; setting up a referrals system between different prescribers to maximise patient benefit; and nurse prescribers mentoring PSP students, and vice versa.

As described earlier, clinical pharmacists were seen as a huge threat to other professionals when they came into hospitals in the 1970s, but their role is now widely accepted. Today, pharmacist prescribers are seen by doctors and nurses as experts in drug therapy but lacking in diagnostic skills and "knowledge" of patients (Buckley *et al.*, 2006). Pharmacist prescribers need to address this actual or perceived lack of "knowledge" of the patient before inter-professional doubts about their prescribing capabilities can be overcome. As stated elsewhere throughout this book, an important factor in designing new roles is having the support of other professional colleagues and patients, and this is what some of the early PSPs have found wanting. There is certainly scope for research into how this can be achieved.

Acknowledgements

I would like to acknowledge the assistance provided by Professor Alison Blenkinsopp and Dr. Janet Grime of Keele University and my pharmacist colleague Paul Buckley.

REFERENCES

Andalo, D. (2003) Community pharmacists decide to 'wait and see' before prescribing. *Prescribing & Medicines Management*, **3**, 5–7.

Avery, A. & Pringle, M. (2005) Extended prescribing by UK nurses and pharmacists. *British Medical Journal*, **331**, 1154–5.

Axon, S. (2003) Is pharmacist prescribing our golden future – or is it a blind alley? *The Pharmaceutical Journal*, **270**, 544.

Britten, N. (2001) Prescribing and the defence of clinical autonomy. *Sociology of Health and Illness*, **23**, 478–96.

Buckley, P., Grime, J. & Blenkinsopp, A. (2006) Inter- and intra-professional perspectives on non-medical prescribing in an NHS trust. *The Pharmaceutical Journal*, **277**, 394–8.

Chen, J. & Britten, N. (2000) 'Strong medicine': an analysis of pharmacist consultations in primary care. *Family Practice*, **17**, 480–3.

Denzin, N. K. & Mettlin, C. J. (1968) Incomplete professionalisation – the case of pharmacy. *Social Forces*, **46**, 375–81.

Department of Health (2005) Nurse and pharmacist prescribing powers extended. Press Release 2005/0395, 10 November. London: Department of Health.

Drug and Therapeutics Bulletin (2006) Non-medical prescribing. *Drugs and Therapeutics Bulletin*, **44**, 33.

Eaton, G. & Webb, B. (1979) Boundary encroachment: pharmacists in a clinical setting. *Sociology of Health and Illness*, **1**, 69–89.

Elston, M. A. (1991) The politics of professional power. In: Gabe, J., Calnan, M. & Bury, M. (eds), *The Sociology of the Health Service*. London: Routledge.

Freeman, G. K., Horder, J. P., Howie, J. G., Hungin, A. P. *et al.* (2002) Evolving general practice consultation in Britain: issues of length and context. *British Medical Journal*, **324**, 880–2

Friedson, E. (1972) *Profession of Medicine: A Study of the Sociology of Applied Knowledge*. New York: Dodd, Mead.

George, J., McCaig, D. J., Bond, C. M., Cunningham, I. T., Diack H. L., Watson A. M. & Stewart, D. C. (2006) Supplementary prescribing: early experiences of pharmacists in Great Britain. *Annals of Pharmacotherapy*, **40**, 1843–5.

Granby, T. (2003) Lessons learnt from the nurse prescribing experience. *Pharmaceutical Journal*, **270**, 24.

Griffiths, M. (2006) Is this the beginning of the end for supplementary prescribing? *Prescribing & Medicines Management*, July edn, 3.

Hughes, C. & McCann, S. (2003) Perceived inter-professional barriers between community pharmacists and GPs. *British Journal of General Practice*, **53**, 600–6.

Lloyd, F., McNally, L. & Hughes, C. M. (2005) Views of hospital nurses/junior house officers/senior house officers on hospital pharmacist supplementary prescribing. *International Journal of Pharmacy Practice*, **13** (Pharmacy Practice Research Supplement), 7.

Lundkvist, J., Akerlind, I., Borgquist, L. & Molstad, S. (2002) The more time spent on listening, the less time spent on prescribing antibiotics in general practice. *Family Practice*, **19**, 638–40.

Martin, C. M., Banwell, C. L., Broom, D. H. & Nisa M. (1999) Consultation length and chronic illness care in general practice: a qualitative study. *Medical Journal of Australia*, **19**(2), 77–81.

McKinlay, J. B. (1977) The business of good doctoring or doctoring as good business: reflections on Friedson's view of the medical game. *International Journal of Health Services*, **3**, 459–83.

Mesler, M. A. (1991) Boundary encroachment and task delegation: clinical pharmacists on the medical team. *Sociology of Health and Illness*, **13**, 310–31.

Turner, B. S. (1987) *Medical Power and Social Knowledge*. London: Sage Publications.

Weiss, M. & Fitzpatrick, R. (1997) Challenges to medicine: the case of prescribing. *Sociology of Health and Illness*, **19**, 297–327.

Professions allied to medicine and prescribing

Alan Borthwick

Although 'prescribing' by non-medically qualified allied health professionals may reasonably be regarded as a recent development in the UK, it is also the case that a small number – most notably podiatrists, optometrists and ambulance paramedics – already enjoy an established history in the legal access, supply, administration and sale of certain restricted medicines (Borthwick, 2001a, 2001b, 2002, 2003, 2004; Borthwick & Nancarrow 2005; Lawrenson, 2005; Titcomb & Lawrenson, 2006). Other allied health professions (AHPs), such as physiotherapy and radiography, developed formal, legal rights to the administration and supply of medicines over a more recent timeframe (Hogg & Hogg, 2006). Across the AHPs, the use of medicines varies; in some cases 'generalist' practitioners may enjoy legal rights to administer, sell and supply restricted medicines, while in other cases it is confined to small numbers working within highly specialised fields (CSP, 1999).

In this chapter, the podiatry, optometry and ambulance paramedical professions serve as useful case exemplars of what might be referred to as early AHP 'prescribing', in the sense of having secured independent, legally acknowledged rights to the access, supply and administration of specific 'prescription only' and 'pharmacy only' medicines some time prior to the availability of 'patient group directions' (PGDs) and 'supplementary' prescribing. Radiography and physiotherapy are included as examples of AHPs that acquired such rights under PGDs and supplementary prescribing. Indeed, within the AHPs there has been a variable degree of interest in pursuing rights to access and administer medicines. 'Early prescribers' such as podiatrists and optometrists arguably sought these legal rights as part of a bid to establish greater autonomy and independence from the medical profession, reflecting perhaps the extent to which these groups operate independently in practice. Others, such as radiography and physiotherapy may have been more accustomed to working as part of a larger healthcare 'team', often in hospital settings, and more readily able, therefore, to accept a medical hierarchy and direction by physicians. Biomedical or clinical scientists, on the other hand, may not require prescribing rights because their roles do not demand direct patient contact. For others, such as occupational or speech and language therapists, the use of medicines may not have traditionally formed part of their therapeutic emphasis or technical repertoire. Optometry, although not strictly classified as an 'allied health profession', nevertheless forms a key example of a non-medical, non-nursing healthcare profession directly involved in the access, supply and administration of restricted medicines and is therefore included in this chapter. Only through an understanding of the earlier 'prescribing' activities of these groups is it possible to evaluate adequately the impact of supplementary prescribing and PGDs on the AHPs as a whole. In this context, 'prescribing' is taken to include the legal right to access, administer, sell and supply specified medicines that are otherwise restricted (that is, those that fall within in the 'prescription only' (POM) and 'pharmacy only' (P) categories of medicine), as well as the actual prescribing inherent in the 'supplementary' and 'independent' forms identified in the Crown Report (DoH, 1999). With the notable exception of ambulance paramedics, all the AHP professions mentioned earlier have recently been granted 'supplementary prescriber' status, with the potential for acquiring 'independent prescriber' status at some time in the future (DoH, 2005; Needle et al., 2007).

At this point, it may be helpful to clarify the way in which AHPs have been accustomed to obtaining and using POM or P medicines prior to supplementary prescribing and patient group directions: they have been 'accessed', 'supplied/sold' and 'administered'. These are important distinctions for understanding the way in which the AHPs have been permitted to obtain, use or sell medicines to patients. In order for an AHP to 'access' a restricted category medicine (and, indeed, to sell, supply and administer it), a legally recognised exemption is required and usually takes the form of a Statutory Instrument. This is a form of 'secondary' legislation and requires the signature of the Health Minister, but not necessarily parliamentary debate, for approval (Adonis, 1993). Statutory Instruments, or 'Orders', allow exemptions to be made to the provisions of a piece of 'primary' legislation (in this case the Medicines Act of 1968), without the need to repeal the Act itself (Adonis, 1993).

Supplying a medicine involves providing it '*directly to a patient or carer for administration*' (DoH, 1999). This must always be undertaken specifically within the course of professional business, as must the 'sale' of a medicine, which generally takes place in the private sector on a fee-for-service basis. Supply involves giving a medicine, in either topical or oral form (e.g. creams, tablets, impregnated dressings or sprays) to the patient or their carer, for the carer to administer or for the patient to self-administer. To 'administer' a medicine is to '*give a medicine either by introduction into the body, whether by direct contact with the body or not, or by external application*' (DoH, 1999). This effectively covers the acts of parenteral administration (i.e. injection of a medicine into the body) or applying dressings which are impregnated with a medicine (which may include 'prescription only' or 'pharmacy only' medicines). For many of the

AHPs, these distinctions illustrate the extent to which the use of medicines is an everyday generalist practice, rather than a specialist activity undertaken by extended-scope practitioners.

In some instances, prior to the advent of patient group directions (DoH, 2000a, 2000b, 2000c), and in the absence of formal statutory exemptions, it has been necessary for physicians to assume overall authority, either by way of specific patient directions or through the operation of 'local agreements' (Freeman, 2006). A degree of latitude has therefore been granted to some AHPs in the absence of legally recognised exemptions, in order to ensure continuity in the patient care pathway.

Medicines and the allied health professions: a brief historical context

It is clear that the crisis in public confidence in healthcare which resulted from the thalidomide tragedy prompted both the Government and the medical profession to review the adequacy of the existing provisions of the medicines legislation as far back as 1962 (BMJ, 1967a, 1967b). As a result, the Government proposed legislation to overhaul existing provisions with new measures controlling the manufacture, quality, testing, marketing, advertising and licensing of medicines, alongside new mechanisms for regulating access, administration, sale and supply (BMJ 1967b; Borthwick, 2001a).

The new Medicines Act (1968) established a Medicines Commission to 'advise Ministers on matters of policy', whose duties would also include the consideration of submissions for exemption by professional groups excluded from rights to access, administer or sell particular medicines falling within the newly established restricted categories (Borthwick 2001a). Under the new classificatory system, medicines were identified as 'Prescription only' (POM), 'pharmacy only' (P) or 'general sales list' (GSL). In particular, 'Prescription only' medicines were accessible only to 'appropriate practitioners' recognised as doctors of medicine, dentists, veterinary surgeons and veterinary practitioners (Medicines Act 1968, Part III). Yet, by 1968, several AHP professions were already accustomed to using a number of medicines which were reclassified under the Act as 'POMs'. New arrangements had to be found to permit them to continue to access and administer these medicines, as well as to make the case for wider exemptions in support of further and future extensions in practice.

By the 1980s, wider political and social changes were influential in ensuring policy reforms gradually made possible an increased access to restricted medicines by the AHPs. In 1985, the Thatcher Government, a conservative administration which espoused a New Right philosophy encouraging the development of market principles within healthcare, introduced a series of reforms which were widely viewed as both anti-monopolistic and anti-professional

(Ham, 1994; Malin Wilmot and Manthorpe, 2002). Among these reforms was the introduction of 'indicative' prescribing, limiting doctors prescribing habits (Bradlow & Coulter, 1993). This was followed shortly thereafter by plans to grant specialist nurses and midwives greater 'prescribing' rights (McCartney *et al.*, 1999; Taylor, 1999).

However, it is worth noting that the move towards prescribing was not a simple step-wise advance. On the contrary, the process involved considerable medical resistance and a significant shift in culture (Borthwick, 2000, 2001a, 2005; McCartney, 1999; Taylor, 1999; Needle *et al.*, 2007). Indeed, the story of AHP 'prescribing' is, in a very real sense, captured cogently and articulately by the neo-Weberian social theorists such as Freidson (1970a, 1970b, 1994, 2001), Abbott (1988) and Larkin (1979, 1980, 1981, 1983, 1988, 1993, 1995) in their use of the explanatory concepts of social closure and medical dominance, illustrating the role of medicine in shaping and constraining paramedical role boundaries.

In 1999, a new trajectory was clearly in evidence, supported by Government policy and captured in the 'Crown Report' review of non-medical prescribing (DoH, 1999). Demographic changes in an ageing population, healthcare recruitment and retention problems and the challenge of EU Working Time Directives limiting doctors' hours all conspired to force a new agenda stressing flexible working and role transfer, primarily from medicine to nursing and the allied health professions (Fournier, 2000; Cameron & Masterson, 2003; Borthwick & Nancarrow, 2005). As a result, the review proposed a radical and novel scenario, in which key nurse and allied health professional groups would emerge as genuine 'prescribers' (DoH, 1999). Two new categories of prescriber were defined – 'independent' and 'dependent' (later 'supplementary'), reflecting the degree of autonomy likely to be bestowed upon those identified as suitable nominees. Five key professional groups were recognised as potential early candidates for independent prescriber status, three of which were AHPs: extended scope physiotherapists; chiropodists and podiatrists; and optometrists (DoH, 1999, para 6.39, page 50). In addition, within a year of the report, the re-formulation of group protocols as 'patient group directions', with legal status, came into effect (DoH, 2000a, 2000b, 2000c).

Podiatry

Podiatry constitutes a useful case study to illustrate the journey of the AHPs towards meaningful 'prescribing' rights. Several phases of regulatory and legislative change established since the Medicines Act of 1968 gradually enabled podiatry to become increasingly recognised as an AHP engaged in the administration, access, supply, and finally prescription of POM and P medicines. These often faltering developments also provide an opportunity to examine the extent to which an expanded range of rights to access medicines has altered practice in an AHP profession. An assessment of the impact of widening access and administration rights in podiatry, alongside the more recent advances in supplementary and, potentially, independent prescribing rights, is possible through an examination of the key shifts in the role and task domains that have evolved over this period, and which are intimately related to, and centrally involved, access to medicines.

Under the Medicines Act (1968), podiatrists were excluded from the provisions relating to 'pharmacy-only' or 'prescription-only' medicines. The immediate impact on podiatry was experienced as a form of deprofessionalisation, in that certain drug preparation practices (mixing agents for topical application), and the use of local anaesthetics by parenteral administration, were no longer to be permitted (Borthwick, 2001a). While it is clear from extant data that relatively few podiatrists did in fact use parenterally administered local anaesthetic agents at this time, the implications for practice were nevertheless clear, and professional autonomy was felt to be acutely undermined (Borthwick, 2000, 2001a, 2005). Approval by the regulatory authority – the Chiropodists Board of the Council for Professions Supplementary to Medicine – was sought in support of the use of local 'analgesic' techniques (that is, the techniques of parenteral injection of these medicines) and was eventually granted in January 1972, after considerable lobbying (Borthwick, 2000, 2001a). However, legislative change was not secured until 1980, when an exemption from Section 58 (2) (b) of the Medicines Act (1968) was eventually signed by the Health Minister, granting access and administration rights to plain solutions of four 'prescription only' injectable local anaesthetic agents (lignocaine hydrochloride, prilocaine hydrochloride, bupivacaine hydrochloride and mepivacaine hydrochloride) (The Chiropodist, 1980).

Access and administration rights to local anaesthetics in particular were important in facilitating a transformation in the role of podiatrists, which required the legal endorsement afforded by the new statutory instrument to fully legitimise practice (Borthwick, 2001b). In fact, a number of statutory instruments at that time gave legal force to the rights of podiatrists to administer, access, supply and sell a range of pharmacy-only medicines (20 in number), as well as the four POM local anaesthetic agents (Borthwick, 2001a).

Local anaesthesia enabled the rapid development of, and extension in, podiatric surgical practice, which would not have been sustainable without established rights to access and administer the necessary medicines (Borthwick, 2005). A variety of surgical techniques were enabled, ranging from toenail avulsions (removals) and hammer toe corrections to more invasive surgical procedures for the correction of hallux valgus (bunions) (Borthwick, 2000, 2005). Local anaesthetic techniques were also rapidly expanded, from ring and infiltration blocks for toe anaesthesia, to ankle block techniques for full foot anaesthesia, enabling more expansive foot surgery. It is still the case today that the majority of podiatric surgical procedures are carried out under local anaesthesia (Borthwick, 2000). Thus, the acquisition of local anaesthetic agents alone enabled a rapid and extensive growth in the scope of practice.

In addition, many of the pharmacy-only agents covered by the new exemption orders permitted podiatrists access to a range of anti-fungal agents such as clotrimazole and miconazole, enabling a more effective clinical approach to dermatophytic infections by generalist podiatrists working in both the NHS and private practice. In the latter case, the capacity to sell these agents to patients was also a significant step forward in providing more comprehensive foot care. Pyrogallol and salicylic acid, as the chemical treatments of choice for managing verrucae, were also included, further legitimising existing therapeutic practices and ending ambiguity over access and administration rights where these medicines were concerned.

Nevertheless, in a changing political climate marked by deregulation and enhanced competition in the provision of healthcare services throughout the 1980s and 1990s, the prospect of further legislative change gained momentum (Borthwick, 1997, 2000, 2001a). By 1994, the Society of Chiropodists and Podiatrists actively sought evidence of 'prescribing' habits among its membership, with a view to developing a further submission. A case was made for access and administration rights to certain oral anti-biotic agents, such as erythromycin, alongside adrenalin for use in emergency circumstances, analgesies for postoperative pain management, and local anaesthetics agents with adrenalin added (JBPM, 1994). Indeed, the Chiropodists Board Medicines Working Party also concluded that evidence from referral patterns for those POM medicines sought (especially anti-biotics) were 'regular' and did merit attention. The Department of Health also published, through the joint NHS Chiropody Task Force document 'Feet First', support for an expanded role for podiatrists in the use of medicines (DoH, 1994). Much attention was given to the way in which such an extension would enable patients to receive more direct and rapid treatment, avoiding duplication of activity and repeated visits to other healthcare professionals (such as GPs). By stressing a streamlined and more direct path for patients to receive the medication required, the logic was designed to appeal to Government policy promoting a seamless, collaborative aproach to care (Borthwick, 2001a).

A new statutory instrument was laid, granting access to some of the requested medicines, but not others – most notably anti-biotics – under the POM (Human Use) Order 1997. Non-steroidal anti-inflammatory drugs (NSAIDs) (ibuprofen and co-dydramol) enabled better pain relief following surgery. Amorolfine was, at the time, a new generation anti-fungal agent, and the addition of adrenalin to the two favoured local anaesthetic agents (lignocaine and bupivacaine) enabled longer anaesthesia for surgery.

The introduction of PGDs in 2000 (and, prior to that, group protocols) enabled podiatrists to access and administer a greater range of medicines. In particular, podiatric surgeons working autonomously within NHS hospital settings were able to use a broad range of medicines, including anti-biotics, powerful analgesics, emergency drugs, anti-emetic agents, anti-coagulants, injectable cortico-steroids and anxiolytics. In doing so, independent provision became increasingly possible, permitting a reduction in duplication of activity and patient referrals (and journeys), appealing directly to the patient-focused agenda so central to the modernisation agenda (NHS Plan, 2001). Other specialist podiatrists working primarily in the fields of hospital-based diabetes care or rheumatology care were also able to obtain a wider range of medicines, circumventing the need to constantly approach physicians for permission to access medicines and allowing the development of new skills in their administration, such as intra-articular injections.

For podiatric surgeons, the advent of group protocols, followed by Patient Group Directions (PGDs), enabled easier access to specific anti-biotics such as gentamicin or fusidic acid in the management of bone infections, or more potent analgesics in the management of post-operative pain. However, it was widely considered that PGDs were limited in that they were unevenly available across the country – in some NHS Trusts PGDs were established with relative ease, in others with great resistance or not at all. Medical hegemony in prescribing was maintained under the system of PGDs, ensuring disparities in access and provision. PGDs were dependent upon a medical sponsor to approve their use, creating occasional problems where role boundary disputes arose. Further policy reforms followed, most visibly through the enactment of the Health and Social Care Act (2001), providing, through section 63, primary legislation enabling non-medical prescribing. This legislation superceded section 58 of the Medicines Act (1968), enabling professionals other than doctors, dentists and veterinarians to attain prescribing rights (nurses having obtained primary legislation earlier, in 1992).

One key difficulty to arise with each approved extension in access and administration was the issue of education and training. The first POM extension for podiatrists relating to POM medicines, in 1980, required a certificate of competence in the use of local anaesthetic agents, attained on successful completion of both written and practical examinations. By the time of the second POM exemption, in 1997, a further upgrading in pharmacology certification was required, which became known colloquially as the 'access and supply', or 'A&S' certificate (SCP, 2006a). Podiatric surgeons already had a separate and extensive training in pharmacology through their surgical training, as part of the fellowship in podiatric surgery, but 'generalist' podiatrists required new courses to accommodate upgrading in tandem with each new provision available. For the most part, only specialist podiatrists were able to access patient group directions, which required specific training and education provisions as part of the approval process, and were, in practice, mainly used by podiatric surgeons.

Specialists in diabetes or rheumatology care (usually self-titled 'diabetes specialist podiatrists' or 'rheumatology specialist podiatrists'), although working in specific areas of care with a high degree of expertise, nevertheless lack specific identifiable credentials in their specialism (Bowen, 2003; Young, 2002, 2003). This anomaly continues to hamper the career progress of these specialists and makes it difficult to draw an objective meaning between 'specialist' and 'generalist' titles (McInnes, 2002). As a result, patient group directions have been rather more problematic and largely dependent upon good relationships with medical staff prepared to endorse an extended repertoire of 'prescribing' to named individuals. In some cases, doctors working in multi-professional team environments such as diabetes care do envisage a wide scope of prescribing for podiatrists, including the treatment and management of hypertension or insulin dose alteration, presumably via supplementary prescribing (Kerr & Richardson, 2000). Similarly, physicians working in rheumatology have expressed supportive views about further extensions in the scope of podiatric rheumatology (Dickson, 1996). However, this is not universal, and the use of PGDs continues to be widely viewed as a temporary measure within podiatric circles until a more satisfactory and clearly acknowledged system is engaged which formalises legitimate prescribing.

To some extent this more formalised process has been established under the guise of 'supplementary prescribing', which was extended to physiotherapists, radiographers and podiatrists in April 2005 (DoH, 2005). Supplementary prescribing, however, requires a significant training and education package, which does not immediately map well to the existing pharmacology programmes provided at undergraduate level. This remains a challenge for educational institutions and their curriculum designers, who must be innovative in moulding existing programmes to accommodate future needs by ensuring the full range of the programme requirements are able to be met. One key advantage will be the stability this will bring to the educational programme, without further need of 'upgrading' every time another statutory instrument granting wider access rights is enacted. Yet, supplementary prescribing has only a limited utility for podiatrists, and there has, to date, been a limited uptake (SCP, 2006b, 2006c, 2007). There are a number of reasons for this. The training for this certification is 'rate limited' in that NHS employers are required to fund and provide the mandatory mentorship associated with the programme, so that the qualification is employer-led (and therefore not available to everyone).

AHP 'supplementary prescribing' also appears to be based on a form of medical delegation, following the specified remit outlined in the clinical management plan, where the AHP assumes the role of monitoring and adjusting existing prescriptions. Most generalist practitioners and all podiatric surgeons work autonomously and independently. Only practitioners specialising in diabetes or rheumatology care and working in hospital (or occasionally community-based) teams are able to adopt supplementary prescribing meaningfully, hence the continued efforts within the profession to attain further access and administration rights via profession-specific Statutory Instruments (SIs), even when supplementary prescribing is available (SCP, 2006c, 2007).

Aside from profession-specific exemptions and the use of PGDs, supplementary and independent prescribing appear at face value to represent the future for AHP prescribing activities. Yet it is only the latter which is regarded as likely to deliver the means by which patient care can be advanced. Indeed, the option most keenly anticipated remains the elusive but much heralded 'independent prescriber' possibility, already granted to pharmacists and nurses, with the AHPs eagerly awaiting the green light to move towards independent prescriber status. However, recent news from the Department of Health suggested that independent prescribing would not be a realistic possibility for the AHPs in 2007, suggesting a 'wait-and-see' policy based on the success of pharmacy and nurse prescribing.

Nevertheless, within podiatry, a recently approved new statutory instrument has extended practice for 'generalists', working in both the NHS and the private sector. It enables suitably qualified practitioners to sell, access and administer an expanded range of POM and P medicines, including the anti-microbials amoxicillin, flucloxacillin and erythromycin, as well as two new generation local anaesthetic agents (ropivacaine and levobupivacaine), adrenalin and methylprednisolone (Medicines for Human Use Order SI 2870/2006). Further 'pharmacy only' additions were also attained, including, for example, the new, highly effective, anti-fungal agent terbinafine.

The real significance of this particular exemption lies in the powers it grants podiatrists to access and sell anti-microbials to combat infections encountered in general practice as well as in specialist care and to access adrenalin for use in emergency circumstances. In the past podiatrists were consistently denied access rights to these medicines, usually justified by reference to concerns over bacterial anti-biotic resistance and fear of overuse (by way of over-prescribing). The change in climate is based on the need to develop a workforce capable of taking on new, expanded roles previously within the exclusive domain of medicine. Again, however, the new extension demands further educational training, although this has been linked to an additional requirement only in terms of immediate life support training for those practitioners currently in possession of the 'A&S' certificate, with a short top-up to the existing pharmacology by way of a focus on anti-biotic therapy. For podiatrists, therefore, there are now several certificated levels at which access and administration of medicines are legally permitted.

Currently, the Society of Chiropodists and Podiatrists is developing a new submission to the Medicines and Healthcare Products Resulatory Agency (MHRA), seeking to gain approval for a further statutory extension which will ensure exclusive access and administration rights for qualified podiatric surgeons to a range of medicines that would not normally be required by podiatrists working in general practice. Because of the specialised nature of the work undertaken by podiatric surgeons, these additional medicines are considered necessary to support good surgical practice. Many of these agents are currently available to podiatric surgeons under PGDs, but these arrangements tend toward regional disparities and lack the autonomy that independent surgical practice demands. The MHRA appears to have recognised this need and has encouraged the SCP to develop further submissions in this way. However, the Health Professions Council, as the regulatory body for the AHPs, has not yet fully developed a sub-specialty register with an accompanying list of recognised 'standards of proficiency', which would acknowledge podiatric surgeons as forming a separate specialty group. Separate recognition would enable them to be distinguished from other practitioners and acknowledged as independent prescribers following the completion of surgical training (SCP, 2007).

Nor are the mechanisms currently in place to enable and expand access and administration rights to the AHPs always seamless in practice. Anomalies occasionally arise and draw attention to unforeseen obstacles or loopholes in the system. Phenol, in its liquefied form, is a highly caustic and erosive chemical, used widely by podiatrists to destroy toenail 'beds', thus preventing re-growth following surgical removal. It is an agent which has been used in practice widely for at least 30 years, with good evidence of its safe handling and effective results (Blake, 2005; Cumming et al., 2005). Only a few years ago, however, it became apparent that this agent does not possess a marketing authorisation (formerly known as a product licence), and is therefore unlicenced.

Authority to use or prescribe unlicensed medicines, under the terms of the Medicines Act (1968), does not extend to AHPs. In spite of long custom and practice, the use of phenol by podiatrists is, strictly speaking, not permitted. A solution appears to have been found, however, in the form of an agent which is now marketed as a medical device and allows phenol to be applied in pharmacologically effective doses for the surgery required, although all other forms of liquefied phenol remain, technically, inaccessible (SCP, 2004).

Optometry

Although documented evidence of the early 'prescribing' activities of optometrists is restricted to a few notable papers authored by Lawrenson (2005) and Titcomb and Lawrenson (2006), supportive accounts from within the profession, alongside a recent Department of Health (2007a) publication and a survey report for the College of Optometrists (2007) enable the construction of a picture which reflects both historical and contemporary practices.

Like podiatry, optometrists have 'traditionally been granted exemptions', which were the only early means of securing change, and these were attained 'sporadically' over a long timeframe (Titcomb & Lawrenson 2006). Key statutory instruments and their additions were secured shortly after the Medicines Act (1968) came into effect, acknowledging optometrists' prior use of medicines. Although predating the Medicines Act (1968), optometrists' use of medicines had been restricted to those employed for diagnostic rather than independent therapeutic purposes, having been largely denied a role in the latter arena under the terms of the Opticians Act (1958) (Larkin, 1981; Lawrenson, 2007). In addition, the lack of regular updating of the early lists of exempted medicines meant that the provisions of the statutory instruments rapidly became dated and, in some cases, irrelevant.

Although the provisions extant in 2004 were said to have been in place since 1978, the key SIs relevant to optometrists relate to the Prescription Only Medicines (Human Use) Order 1997 (the POM Order), the Medicines (Pharmacy and General Sale-Exemption) Order 1980 and the Medicines (Sale or Supply) (Miscellaneous Provisions) Regulations 1980 (MHRA, 2004). For example, the pre-2005 POM list included medicines such as the anti-muscarinic agent hyoscine, the non-steroidal anti-inflammatory drug oxyphenbutazone and the miotic agents bethanechol, neostigmine and physostigmine, which, years before the 2005 amendment, were no longer commercially available for use by optometrists in the UK (Titcombe & Lawrenson, 2006). Similarly, as in the case of other AHPs, access to anti-bacterial anti-biotic agents for supply or sale was resisted (see Freidson, 1970b, for an account of the importance of prescribing to medical authority and hegemony in healthcare). Initially only sulphacetamide, and later chloramphenicol, were permitted, and the sole alternative – framycetin sulphate – was limited to 'administration' use only and therefore not accessible for supply purposes.

These restrictions clearly curtailed the therapeutic interventions of optometrists in the years following the Medicines Act (1968), limiting existing practice and preventing further developments which would enhance the therapeutic role of the optometrist. Indeed, the key problem with the medicines list exemptions was that they contained primarily drugs essential to the diagnostic process and included fewer medicines for therapeutic use (SCP, 2006b). For example, chloramphenicol was the sole anti-biotic agent available for sale or supply to patients with superficial eye infections or for use as a prophylactic measure to guard against infection following an ocular surface injury. Indeed, it was not generally used therapeutically because optometrists were required to refer such patients to ophthalmologists (Larkin, 1981, 1983; Lawrenson, 2007). Framycetin sulphate, which might have better served these purposes, was limited to 'administration' use only, rendering it unhelpful in the full management of eye infections, as the patient could not be supplied with the medicine over the necessary time frame to adequately eliminate the infection. Repeated visits to the optometrist to have the drug administered would not have been feasible, given that the treatment might require several applications daily for a period of several days.

Indeed, prior to 2005, when significant changes to optometrist 'prescribing' took effect, the profession was limited to chloramphenicol in eye-drop form (at no greater than 0.5%) and eye ointment preparations (no greater than 1%) for sale or supply. The only other POM agents made available were from a range of 14 anti-inflammatory, miotic and anti-muscarinic agents similar to those previously mentioned. In terms of administration, the list was restricted to the anti-biotic framycetin and a number of local anaesthetic agents, such as amethocaine, lignocaine, oxybuprocaine and proxymetacaine hydrochlorides, and anti-inflammatory agents, such as oxyphenbutazone. In 2005, however, access, administration, sale and supply rights were expanded and supplementary prescribing rights introduced (Needle *et al.*, 2007). The former consisted of an updated list of POM agents made available to all currently registered optometrists.

In addition, a relaxation in the regulations surrounding the supply of 'pharmacy only' and general sales list (GLS) agents, coupled with the establishment of a further list of POM medicines to be made available to optometrists with 'extended training', was introduced (Titcomb & Lawrenson, 2006).

Supplementary prescribing rights were granted to suitably qualified optometrists as part of the wider programme of health policy reform on extended AHP roles (DoH, 2000, 2001). The rationale behind the extended list centred on removing six medications from the existing lists because they were no longer commercially available, and replacing framycetin with fusidic acid. Fusidic acid would be made available for supply and sale as well as administration, by way of a written order for presentation to a pharmacist (negating, therefore, the limitation requiring sale and supply in emergency circumstances only) (Needle *et al.*, 2007). Removing this limitation was viewed as important because it was felt to be 'unnecessarily restrictive in today's climate' (Titcomb & Lawrenson, 2006). Indeed, optometrists commonly store a range of ocular lubricants for supply purposes, many of which have been reclassified as 'devices', which, under previous legislation, were deemed to be available for supply in emergency circumstances only (Titcomb & Lawrenson, 2006).

Optometrists are now able to supply any relevant 'pharmacy only' agent, including lubricants, anti-allergy preparation and anti-microbials, effectively placing them on a par with pharmacists in the access of required P medicines (Titcomb & Lawrenson, 2006). In addition, a change in the wording of the Opticians Act (21958) was enabled in 2000, effectively allowing optometrists greater freedom to undertake a therapeutic role (Lawrenson, 2007).

A further list of new medicines was granted for specialist optometrists registered as such with the General Optical Council, following specialist training (Titcomb & Lawrenson, 2006). This enables a broader range of healthcare interventions by specialist optometrists, notably in many common, non-sight threatening ocular disorders such as infective and allergic conjunctivitis, blepharitis, 'dry eye' and superficial injury. Within the SI, the additional POM list is indicated as 'additional supply', and the eligible optometrists are referred to as 'additional supply optometrists', distinguishing them from generalist optometrists, who are excluded from this provision. Thus, there are now two levels of exemption within optometry – one for 'entry-level' optometrists, such a new graduates or existing general optometry practitioners, and a second, specialist level for postgraduate trained optometrists, which includes further anti-microbials, musolytic, anti-histamine and mast cell stabilising agents (Titcomb & Lawrenson, 2006).

Nonetheless, there are drawbacks. Even specialist optometrists, with the extended lists available to them, cannot prescribe any alternative to medications with anti-microbial preservatives should allergic responses to the preservatives arise, although symptomatic treatment in the form of sodium diclofenac is available. Specialist optometrists undergo a 2-year training programme in the theory and practice of prescribing, which, like the more generic supplementary prescribing curricula developed by the AHP Supplementary Prescribing Steering Group (guided by the competency framework devised by the National Prescribing Centre), includes a 'learning in practice' element. It currently consists of 5 days of placement with a medical mentor in a hospital ophthalmology department (Titcomb & Lawrenson, 2006). Furthermore, some of the agents included in the 2005 lists are now also redundant, demonstrating sharply the limitations of this type of legislative means of enabling 'prescribing'. Production of polymyxin B and bacitracin was discontinued in early 2005, as it was for thymoxamine, an alpha-adrenoreceptor blocker. New anti-histamines were launched after the consultation period and are not included in the lists. The additional training requirements for 'additional supply list' practitioners are, however, broadly considered to be excessive, with only 200 trained optometrists reported in 2007 (Needle *et al.*, 2007).

Supplementary prescribing offers many of the same advantages to optometrists as it has to the other recipients of this status. It is felt to be 'most useful when dealing with long-term medical conditions', which, for optometrists, largely means the management of glaucoma (Titcomb & Lawrenson, 2006). It may also have a role in post-surgical management, such as following cataract or refractive surgery, where pain relief, anti-microbial prophylaxis and treatment of infections are relevant. Optometrists, however, were identified as possible early candidates for independent prescribing, and there is broad support within the profession for this version of prescribing to be made available. Supplementary prescribing, although helpful in certain circumstances, is widely viewed as relevant only to practitioners working within healthcare teams, for example, in hospital ophthalmology clinics, and much less applicable to the majority of practitioners working within their own practices in the community and in the private sector. (Needle *et al.* found that over 90% of study respondents were community-based.)

Much of optometry is, of necessity, involved in retail business, and the majority of the professional's profit is derived from sales of optical devices – spectacles and contact lenses – rather than the sale of professional services. In these circumstances, there are few incentives to adopt the new role of supplementary prescriber because of the lack of extra remuneration, fear of litigation and the considerable training time and costs (Needle *et al.*, 2007). A further barrier remains the 'frequency and quality of referral feedback' from medical practitioners, evidently more problematic with ophthalmologists than GPs (Needle *et al.*, 2007). Currently, the Department of Health is undertaking a public consultation on the introduction of independent prescribing for optometrists, a move which would be welcomed by the profession and may help to circumvent many of the obstacles noted here (Titcomb & Lawrenson, 2006; Needle *et al.*, 2007).

Ambulance paramedics

Interestingly, although ambulance paramedics have been involved both formally and informally in the access and administration of medicines for many years, these practices have been largely ignored in the healthcare literature. Accounts from within the profession constitute the basis of the picture portrayed here of early involvement in the access and administration of medicines.

It appears clear that, prior to the 1970s, ambulance paramedics enjoyed no specific rights to either the access or administration of medicines from the restricted POM categories described under the Medicines Act (1968). Nevertheless, they were able to be 'certificated' in the administration of oxygen and nitrous oxide gases. Indeed, the administration of intravenous fluids (not containing POM medicines) was a practice common throughout the 1970s and formed a core part of paramedical practice. The NHS reorganisation of 1974, resulting in a vast expansion in the provision of services within a reconfigured structure of Regional Health Authorities and Area Health Authorities, saw the amalgamation of hospital and community services as part of a bid to ensure greater integration and effectiveness (Ham, 1994; Webster, 2002). For the ambulance service, this meant full integration into the NHS, as, prior to 1974, many services had been delivered by Local Borough Councils.

Paramedical practice, by its nature, often involved working independently from the medical profession. The use of patient-specific directions was not a feasible option, and authority to carry out many of the activities involving administration of medicines had to be secured through other, formal mechanisms, although these were not supported by legal exemption Orders. One such example was the use of Paramedical Steering Groups set up within the Health Authority ambulance service structure. Strict protocols were devised to ensure good practice and clear guidance to paramedics in the field, and authority to carry out procedures involving the administration of medicines (such as the POM adrenalin) was achieved through a 'blanket' coverage granted by the presiding medical consultant sitting on the Steering Group. This 'cover' was provided on a condition-specific basis, enabling ambulance paramedics to operate with some freedom within a strictly codified set of circumstances.

Ambulance paramedics did, however, succeed in securing, along with podiatry and optometry, a statutory exemption – the Prescription Only Medicines (Human Use) Order 1997 (SI 1997/ 1830) – permitting access and administration rights to a range of medicines. Administration rights for medicines given by an intravenous route, such as adrenalin in emergency life-saving circumstances, and diazepam for sedation, essentially gave legal cover for existing, core practices. It also provided paramedics with the right to administer glucose, the anti-coagulant agent heparin and local anaesthetic agents such as lignocaine hydrochloride.

More recently, the Department of Health has approved a series of PGDs for ambulance paramedics for use in 'mass casualty situations' for which 'chemical and biological countermeasures' may become necessary (e.g. DoH, 2007b). Despite attempts by the British Paramedic Association to ensure the inclusion of paramedics as candidates for AHP supplementary prescribing, the profession has not yet been granted this status (Furber, 2007, pers. comm.).

Radiography

Although radiographers have, like podiatrists, optometrists and ambulance paramedicals, an established history in the administration of medicines, until the advent of PGDs these activities lacked legal status and often operated through local protocols (Hogg & Hogg, 2006). Intravenous administration of contrast agents, radiopharmaceuticals and adjunct drugs such as buscopan were common practice 'for many years, perhaps decades' (Hogg & Hogg, 2006).

In some circumstances, for example, when drug administration was 'time-critical', the direct involvement of the radiographer was an essential element in the smooth running of radiological services. In services such as renography, diuretic administration by radiographers became central to the effective functioning of the service provision. Some of these practices may have been enabled through the use of patient-specific directions, in which a radiologist might write an instruction on a patient request form, but in many instances the radiographer worked without such specific written instructions (Freeman, 2006). Clearly, some of these practices lacked the endorsement of strict legality, in the absence of any statutory exemption, effectively meaning that 'some of this early practice broke the law' (Hogg & Hogg, 2006). Anecdotal evidence from within the profession suggests that some of these practices continue today, for example, when radiographers may not always be aware of the legal status of contrast agents (Freeman, 2007, pers. comm.).

By 2003, in the wake of the Crown Report (DoH, 1999), the Society and College of Radiographers had identified a number of key areas of radiographic practice for which 'prescribing' would be relevant. These included radiotherapy, contrast radiography, renography and the use of radiopharmaceuticals, and viewed prescribing as 'not an option for the future . . . [but] a requirement' (CoR, 2001; Freeman, 2006; Hogg & Hogg, 2003). In addition, it was recognised that differences in specialist skills and working practices would ensure the need for both supplementary and independent versions of prescribing, as in specialist areas such as radiotherapy radiography, sonography, gastrointestinal radiography and nuclear medicine radiography (Hogg & Hogg, 2003). Indeed, many specialist radiographers undertake activities requiring the administration of medicines in a fairly autonomous pattern, as noted in a college report on role development (CoR, 1996), which specified intravenous injections, barium enema examinations and patient review clinics (SCoR, 2002).

Authority for these activities has often been 'delegated' to the radiographer through 'local agreements and schemes of work', regarded as a less than satisfactory position (SCoR, 2002). The SCoR report (2002), written in response to the Crown Report (DoH, 1999), also identified a comprehensive list of 'broad categories' of clinical expertise for which prescribing might be expected to be directly relevant for radiographers. Most notable were the areas of bone densitometry, computerised tomography and gastro-intestinal work requiring the use of contrast agents. It also included interventional angiography, magnetic resonance imaging, mammography, nuclear medicine and oncology treatment related toxicity. While the report supported access to 'the entire formulary', an approved indicative list of medicines was included, covering 12 radioisotopes, 10 radiopharmaceuticals, barium products, iodine-based contrast agents and gas-producing agents for internal gastro-intestinal work. It also noted the use of chemical reagents, as well as a vast array of medical devices such as fertility thermometers, incontinence appliances and pessaries.

In relation to oncology care, the list was extensive, and included NSAIDs such as ibuprofen, co-codamol and co-proxamol for pain relief, as well as bisacodyl and other agents for managing constipation. Furthermore, steroid creams were considered important for managing irradiated skin, and anti-microbial agents (such as acyclovir, nystatin and chlorhexidene) in the management and prevention of infections. Drugs for treating diarrhoea, related rectal symptoms, nausea and vomiting were featured as part of the management of treatment side effects.

Within nuclear medicine, anti-biotics such as trimethoprim and Coamoxiclav (combining amoxicillin with clavulanic acid in managing bacterial resistance) were identified as necessary adjuncts to effective practice. So, too, were captopril (an angiotensin-converting enzyme inhibitor), cimetidine (in ulcer management) and phenobarbitone barbiturates. Each specialty area had a specific range of medicines identified, and even 'generalist' practice was felt to merit access to anti-spasmodic medication, and, very rarely, to anti-biotics such as gentamycin and amoxicillin for prophylactic use prior to barium enema.

However, undergraduate pharmacology education was variable between different higher education institutions (HEI) (SCoR, 2002). Indeed, Freeman (2006) pointed to the fact that 'there is no specific training that radiographers must undertake before they are able to work under a PGD' because PGDs do not specify a particular educational programme in pharmacology. Yet as early as 1993, a national survey of advanced practice was conducted within the specialty of nuclear medicine and found that 74% of radiographers were administering diagnostic radiopharmaceuticals (with 14% using therapeutic radiopharmaceuticals) (Hogg & Hogg, 2006).

Hogg and Hogg (2006) also claimed that it was likely that 'administrations during the 1980s were related to radiopharmaceuticals and the growth in the 1990s was related to x-ray contrast media', reflecting the evolving and expanding role boundaries within radiography. By 2006, it was also clear that the educational benchmark statements for radiography required undergraduate education to address the issues of 'understanding methods of administration of contrast agents and drugs, including intravenous administration'. In 2001, the College of Radiographers recognised the need to adapt undergraduate education to include relevant pharmacology and to dovetail this with appropriate and relevant postgraduate education in support of further prescribing in specialist fields (CoR, 2001). One suggestion was to incorporate into undergraduate programmes a framework of education in pharmacology that would enable graduates to work as supplementary prescribers, leaving postgraduate education to focus on specialist areas in which a radiographer might become an independent prescriber (CoR, 2001). A new 'learning and development framework' document (to be published) by the College of Radiographers, establishes the requirement that all new undergraduate course approvals will have to include pharmacology programmes, although the practical use of pharmaceuticals will still largely occur at a postgraduate level (Freeman, 2007, pers. comm.). This approach is already evident in the approved certification of competence in administering intravenous injections, for which the academic component is completed during the course and the practical element completed under supervision within six months thereafter (Freeman, 2006).

Prior to the introduction of supplementary prescribing for radiographers in 2005, PGDs, available from 2000, became the principle means of securing legal cover for the administration of, and access to, POM and P medicines. Many radiographers utilised group protocols prior to PGDs to enable the supply and administration of medicines (CoR, 2001; Synergy News, 2006a). Indeed, since 1998 radiographers deploying group protocols (and subsequently PGDs) were in receipt of postgraduate level training in pharmacology (Francis and Hogg, 2006). By 2006, the most commonly used medicines under PGD for diagnostic radiographers included contrast agents, laxatives, sodium chloride and local topical anaesthetics. Less common activities such as adenosine stress testing in nuclear cardiology are also now part of the remit for radiographers.

For therapeutic radiographers, the most common agents specified in PGDs have been NSAIDs for pain relief and rectal symptoms, as well as medication for constipation, diarrhoea and wound care (Hogg & Hogg, 2006). A cited example in which PGDs are used in oncology radiography highlights the relatively seamless care attained; in this case a radiographer assessed, advised upon and supplied pre-packs of Imodium to patients experiencing diarrhoea following pelvic radiotherapy, with the clear benefit of avoiding reliance on time-consuming referral to the oncologist (Francis & Hogg, 2006). PGDs have also been thought to enable radiographers to work with a degree of independence from doctors within the cancer care setting, particularly when the supply of medicines is concerned (Kirkbride & Craig, 2006).

It has certainly been noted in the literature that the evolving role of the radiographer has often been 'constrained by the radiographer's inability to prescribe drugs for the management of treatment toxicity' in the arena of oncology care (Francis & Hogg, 2006). In some instances, the skills of the radiographer have not been fully utilised as a result of these limitations, when 'radiographers could provide a better service' (Shepherd, 2000). Indeed, Shepherd (2000) has even suggested that the future role of the radiotherapy radiographer may come to involve chemotherapy administration.

In this context, supplementary prescribing has been viewed as 'both exciting and demanding', and for radiographers working in oncology care, it is felt to be 'most useful for chronic conditions, for example, the cancer disease trajectory which involves significant extended periods of care following initial diagnosis' (Francis & Hogg, 2006). Experience of the use of PGDs has indicated certain drawbacks for radiographers, with a low rate of use following completion of the postgraduate training. Lack of 'whole-hearted' support for mentoring by physicians has been a common experience, and the success of supplementary prescribing will also hinge on these requirements (Francis & Hogg, 2006). 'Working patterns with PGDs' suggest that relatively few radiographers will continue to use PGDs simply to facilitate advanced practice and are more likely to deploy them within 'radiographer-led treatment reviews' (Francis & Hogg, 2006).

Integrated care may be best served by ensuring that sufficient numbers of radiographic supplementary prescribers are made available on each treatment unit. This would help to ensure that a 'single' prescriber would not be employed across a number of units merely as a resource to be used to 'purely . . . prescribe for the side effects' of patient treatments, a scenario which it is felt may lead to a rise in 'tension' within radiography teams (Francis and Hogg, 2006).

Furthermore, PGDs also demand regular updating, particularly when the drug product characteristic changes. The process of updating can be slow and subject to delays, taking 'days at best, months at worst' to renew or upgrade (Hogg & Hogg, 2006). If the drug product characteristic does change, the PGD 'could become obsolete overnight', effectively requiring a suspension in the related activities of the radiographer until the PGD is upgraded to incorporate the change. Hogg and Hogg (2006) consider the benefit of supplementary prescribing, in this context to rest with the greater freedom to adapt to such events alongside a reduction in the related paperwork. Because the clinical management plan underpinning supplementary prescribing does not need to be drug-specific, unlike a PGD, there is greater flexibility and applicability, permitting a drug change when necessary.

Freeman (2006) also considered supplementary prescribing to be a useful option for therapeutic radiographers when 'working in on-treatment review may . . . smooth the patient pathway'. Saving time and easing the patient journey are central to the arguments in favour of supplementary prescribing in the context of integrated care, for which 'it has got to be helpful not to be passed on to another practitioner to get a prescription for, say, pain relief' (Evans, 2004).

The growth in scope of practice in radiography has been highlighted by the advent of 'consultant radiographer' grades within the NHS, in which effectively autonomous practitioners may need to assume responsibility for a caseload in a specialist field. In the first such case, a consultant therapy radiographer specialising in lung palliative care assumed the responsibility for prescribing patients radiotherapy regimes (Synergy News, 2003). Also, in the field of oncology palliative care, the first 'trainee consultant radiographer' scheme was launched in 2006, involving a 2-year training programme leading to consultant status in which the practitioner should become clinical lead in both palliative radiotherapy and supplementary prescribing (Synergy News, 2006b). Supplementary prescribing (SP) has been considered 'well suited' to the work undertaken by therapy radiographers, and may be preferable to PGDs because the latter are restricted to specific medicines at specific dosages. No such constraint applies in supplementary prescribing, enabling the therapy radiographer to offer 'more responsive and 'more individualised care' (Hogg et al., 2007).

Yet supplementary prescribing may, in turn, present the radiographer with a number of challenges. For example, one of the requirements of supplementary prescribing is that a specific diagnosis should have been concluded prior to proceeding with the clinical management plan. If this demand is strictly observed, then, as Hogg and Hogg (2006) point out, 'it goes without saying' that supplementary prescribing may be of 'limited clinical use' in diagnostic radiography, as much of the work is designed to establish a diagnosis. It is also unclear how supplementary prescribing will work in certain instances. For example, some cancers requiring radiography interventions may be regarded as 'long-term' conditions, with life expectancy extended for many years. If patients return with a recurrence after a gap of a year, will supplementary prescribing under the existing clinical management plan still be possible (Freeman, 2007, pers. comm.)? A similar point is raised by Hogg et al. (2007), when evaluating the applicability of supplementary prescribing in diagnostic radiography. In the example cited, diagnostic radiographers may occasionally undertake serial imaging in nuclear medicine and bone densitometry, possibly over several years (in cancer imaging). However, the frequency of such serial imaging may be less than once a year, and the clinical management plan must be reviewed annually (Hogg *et al.*, 2007). For the most part, diagnostic imaging involves 'one-off examinations', which are usually completed within 6 hours, to which supplementary prescribing would not be relevant (Hogg *et al.*, 2007).

Hogg and Hogg (2006) also express some concern over the way some PGDs are currently being used by radiographers. In noting that a recent survey of advanced practitioner gastro-intestinal radiographers revealed a certain lack of knowledge about the use and application of PGDs, they highlight one example in which an existing PGD utilises, in effect, off-licence use when this is justified by suggesting the practice is 'supported by national practice' (Hogg & Hogg, 2006).

As far as diagnostic radiography is concerned, the continuing use of PGDs and the prospect of independent prescribing may be more relevant than supplementary prescribing. In some cases, for example, in skin or oral care, departments operating with PGDs which were established prior to the availability of supplementary prescribing are often felt to be preferable, in spite of their disadvantages (Freeman, 2007, pers. comm.). At the time of writing, only one diagnostic radiographer was known to be undertaking a supplementary prescribing course, and the College of Radiographers has expressed the view that without independent prescriber status, many radiographers will continue to experience departmental 'bottlenecks' in which delays are caused by the ongoing need to ensure direct physician involvement (Freeman, 2007, pers. comm.).

It is possible that the use of independent prescribing by diagnostic radiographers might follow a pattern already identified by Hogg and Hogg (2006) as part of current practice in accident centres in which radiographers are involved in supplying discharged patients with analgesics such as ibuprofen. In this situation, the radiographer is considered to be engaged in establishing a diagnosis, devising a management plan and enacting a discharge with (or without) medication and does so currently under PGD (Hogg *et al.*, 2007). For Hogg and Hogg (2006), this aspect of the radiographer role is consistent with the activities of an independent prescriber, as defined in the Crown Report (DoH, 1999), and provides a justification for a move towards independent radiography prescribing.

Physiotherapy

Prescribing activity within physiotherapy has been a comparatively recent development, and one firmly linked to specialist 'extended scope practitioner' levels of practice (DoH, 1999). Currently there is no pharmacology component within the undergraduate educational programme, although postgraduate education has been extended to accommodate supplementary prescribing since 2005 (DoH, 2005; Oxlade, 2006).

Prior to the advent of supplementary prescribing, physiotherapists involved in the access and administration of medicines were largely limited to those working within the musculo-skeletal arena. Central to this role was the use of 'injection therapy' techniques, consisting of the intra-articular or soft-tissue delivery of cortico-steroid agents. These agents are used primarily by physiotherapists for the suppression of inflammation and pain relief in acute, mainly soft tissue, inflammatory disorders.

Until the legislation enabling the use of PGDs and supplementary prescribing was introduced, however, the profession had no specific statutory instruments granting exemptions from the terms of the Medicines Act (1968). When the administration of a medicine was undertaken prior to the use of group protocols, the only available means of ensuring legal practice was to operate within the patient-specific directions of a physician. As a result, close working relationships with medical professionals have usually been something of a pre-requisite for such practices. By 2003 it was acknowledged that 'a large number' of physiotherapists utilised PGDs, although it was noted that 'there are also a number who do not and should be doing so', implying that the mechanism might be used more widely than was actually the case (CSP, 2003).

Injection therapy, as a central component of specialist physiotherapy practice, largely involves 'short-term' treatments for soft-tissue complaints such as 'tennis elbow', De Quervain's tenosynovitis, plantar fasciitis and, to a lesser extent, carpal tunnel syndrome, in which injections are delivered regularly over a period of days, weeks or months (CSP, 1999). In addition, corticosteroid 'injection' therapy is helpful in managing overuse and athletic injuries (CSP, 1999). The evidence is more equivocal for cortico-steroid use in intra-articular administration for the management of pain in osteoarthritis, although pain reduction in cases of inflammatory rheumatoid arthritis may be helpful. Physiotherapists may also use local anaesthetic agents, often in combination with injectable cortico-steroids, giving a relatively small range of specific medications for use within a narrow spectrum of extended scope specialist practice. In most instances, the range of injectable medicines is limited to hydrocortisone acetate, triamcinoline acetonide or hexacetonide, and methylprednisolone acetate, alongside the local anaesthetic lignocaine (usually without the addition of adrenalin).

As late as 1996, a statement from the Medical Defence Union, included in the Chartered Society of Physiotherapists guidelines on injection therapy (CSP, 1999), referred to the legal provisions at the time, in which 'the doctor will be clinically responsible for the prescription, and the physiotherapist will be administering the injections in accordance with the directions of the doctor', illustrating the extent to which physiotherapy 'prescribing' practices were reliant upon medical supervision. However, since 2000, the increasing use of PGDs and the advent of supplementary prescribing has witnessed a new breadth to the involvement of physiotherapists in the use of POM and 'pharmacy-only' medicines. While the musculo-skeletal speciality probably represents the area most involved in the access, administration and supply of medicines currently, and remains the area likely to form the vanguard in the push for an exemption Order (as suggested by the CSP Steering Group on Prescribing), other speciality areas have emerged as potential prescriber groups.

Supplying anti-inflammatory agents and non-opioid analgesics is already a feature of physiotherapy supplementary prescribing practice, and the management of acute or chronic 'spinal' pain has been considered (Limb, 2006). In addition, it has been suggested that physiotherapists working in neuro-rehabilitation have a 'strong role' to play in the use of anti-spasticity medication, using botulinum toxin, and that respiratory physiotherapists may become involved in the prescription and supply of bronchodilators (Limb, 2006). It has also been suggested that physiotherapists might, in due course, become involved in prescribing anti-cholinergic drugs for 'over-active bladder symptoms' in the emergent specialist area of 'women's health' (Limb, 2006). However, for the most part, access and administration of POM medicines within physiotherapy practice is confined to the musculo-skeletal specialty, and drug administration is achieved mainly by parenteral routes. In the majority of instances, these are covered under patient group directions in the NHS workplace, although a growing number of physiotherapists working in the private sector face a more difficult challenge in accessing and administering POM agents.

Physiotherapists in the private sector are increasingly finding themselves in a position where, although highly trained in injection therapy techniques, they do not have rights to administer the required POM medicine (PGDs do not apply outside the NHS). For example, if a patient with a soft-tissue injury is deemed likely to benefit therapeutically from a course of parenterally administered methylprednisolone acetate by a physiotherapist working independently in the private sector, the therapist does not have the legal right to administer the medicine although he or she may be certificated and approved by the professional body in the techniques of soft-tissue injection. What is required in order to enable the therapist to work within the provisions of the Medicines Act (1968), in the absence of exemptions, is a patient-specific direction from a physician. While this may be forthcoming, it is unlikely that the therapist will receive written instruction in every case. This constitutes a significant obstacle to autonomous physiotherapy practice, and no obvious alternative is as yet evident other than via the route of supplementary prescribing, although it is unclear how even this might operate in the circumstances outlined here.

Many physiotherapists continue to work independently, in the private sector, utilising local agreements with GPs to sustain injection therapy practices, although this is widely felt to be unsatisfactory. The CSP has expressed support for supplementary prescribing as a means of enhancing care in long-term chronic conditions, but views independent prescribing as more likely to be relevant for acute musculo-skeletal work, and this would also apply to the private sector (Frontline, 2004). Nevertheless, supplementary prescribing has been considered relevant even in circumstances in which physiotherapists work in 'remote locations' in community settings without immediate recourse to a physician, although mainly for dosage alteration under an established clinical management plan (Limb, 2005, 2006). In a recent example of AHP prescribing practices at specialist level, a physiotherapy consultant in intermediate care, leading an inter-disciplinary team involved in elderly rehabilitation, was called upon to prescribe a range of POM and P medicines. In this case, the prescribing span included analgesics for use in pain relief, anti-coagulants in cardiovascular prophylaxis and anti-biotic anti-microbial management of methicillin resistant staphylococcal infections (Limb, 2006).

Conclusion

To convey an appropriate and informed account of AHP prescribing, it has been necessary to consider the range of means by which medicines are accessed and deployed in practice. To address only the supplementary prescribing initiative would fail to do justice to the AHPs and their broad use of medicines. In this light, supplementary prescribing represents one step in an ongoing process which continues to unfold, shaped by a complex web of social, political and cultural changes. Although perhaps too early to judge, it appears that supplementary prescribing is of limited utility and applicability for some in the AHPs, and, in certain respects, may reflect the continuing dominance of medicine in determining the degree and extent of AHP prescribing.

Many AHPs rely on a range of tools to access medicines, including supplementary prescribing, PGDs and profession specific statutory instruments, with every indication that they will continue to do so. No one mechanism has, as yet, proved more popular than another, although, in general, independent prescribing is felt likely to offer the best option in future, especially for specialist, consultant AHP practitioners. There is little doubt that enhanced or new prescribing roles for the AHPs will enable greater independence in practice and a more comprehensive approach to patient care. Restricted or absent prescribing rights has, in the past, been a significant obstacle to effective practice for many of the AHPs, requiring unnecessary reliance on physician involvement when carrying out tasks in which the practitioner is already often skilled, competent and experienced. It is, perhaps, because of the broad concern expressed by the medical profession that further expansion is slow. An underpinning appreciation and detailed understanding of the physiological and pharmacological effects of medicines, and their associated complications, is clearly regarded as a necessary pre-requisite to prescribing. However, current education and training in this field is widely held to be robust and carefully monitored, offering concrete assurances that eligible candidates are adequately prepared.

The concern that an enhanced prescribing authority for the AHPs might unleash a wave of over-prescribing has not in any way yet materialised. When it already forms an integral part of practice, prescribing has simply enabled more coherent, seamless practice, by virtue of the freedom to operate unhindered by the need to constantly refer (or defer) to medical authority. Where it is new, it is proving helpful in ensuring greater responsiveness to patient need, and constitutes a useful exemplar of flexible working, which lies at the heart of contemporary healthcare policy and workforce planning. AHPs appear to be utilising prescribing authority in a measured and coherent fashion. When it is necessary for practice, it is adopted. When it is unnecessary, it is avoided. Perhaps a review of all existing instances of the use of patient-specific directions, in which the physician directs an AHP to undertake some prescribing activity, would demonstrate those areas where further autonomous prescribing should be considered. Effective and safe practice is evidenced by the extensive use of PGDs or statutory exempted lists by certain AHP professionals, such as podiatric surgeons or additional supply optometrists, and this suggests a clear case for independent prescribing in these instances.

Currently, there are 13 AHPs registered with the Health Professions Council. In addition to those already featured in this chapter, these include art therapists, biomedical scientists, clinical scientists, dieticians, occupational therapists, operating department practitioners, orthoptists, speech and language therapists and prosthetists and orthotists. Of the total, nine already enjoy, or have been directly considered for, prescribing privileges in one form or another. It is intriguing to consider which other AHPs may, in due course, join them.

Recent legislation permits the use of PGDs by dieticians, occupational therapists, orthoptists, prosthetists and orthotists and speech and language therapists, giving some indication of the trend towards prescribing within the wider AHP community. It may be possible to predict that some AHPs, such as art therapists, would be unlikely prescribers, bearing in mind their use of art or music therapy as an effective alternative to pharmacological therapy. Certainly, clinical psychologists appear to have largely eschewed the opportunity to become involved as prescribers, preferring instead to focus, like art and music therapists, on alternative, non-pharmacological therapeutic strategies. On the other hand, operating department practitioners (ODPs), dieticians and speech and language therapists are already engaging in activities which would be fruitfully enhanced by greater access to prescribing privileges. To some extent this is evident from the literature, which continues to highlight emergent role boundary disputes between professions working in related fields, such as in operating theatre protocols, for which the handling of controlled drugs remains a contested area between ODPs and theatre nurses (see Timmons & Tanner, 2004). Such data suggest that an extension in prescribing rights to ODPs would be both welcome and timely.

It is also a striking indicator of need that some AHPs continue to seek further exemptions, under statutory instrument, in spite of the availability of PGDs and supplementary prescribing. Currently the Society of Chiropodists and Podiatrists and the Chartered Society of Physiotherapists are seeking to expand (podiatrists) and create (physiotherapists) lists which will better serve the needs of podiatric surgeons and extended scope physiotherapists respectively, the former seeking an extensive 'second-level' list, the latter a small but select list. Supplementary prescribing courses for the AHPs are now emerging across the country, often jointly validated with nurse supplementary prescribing programmes. Recent data from the HPC website indicate that, to date, 35 supplementary prescribing courses have been approved, delivered at 30 different higher education institutions (HEIs) (HPC, 2007).

AHP prescribing offers many benefits to the professions and their patients and enhances the quality of healthcare provision. Faster, more accessible care for patients is a clear advantage. Easing the patient pathway and ensuring the appropriate medication is provided in a timely manner constitutes a major benefit and is an asset to the service. Role transfer has enabled allied health professionals to expand their therapeutic repertoire, deepen their knowledge, and enhance their overall contribution to healthcare. Greater coherence in the delivery of care has been enabled, in tandem with the shifting spheres of practice in a changing workforce.

To date, few disadvantages have emerged, other than the slow uptake of supplementary prescribing opportunities by some AHPs. Without doubt this relates to the lack of perceived relevance and applicability of this form of prescribing, rather than a reluctance to undergo further training or assume wider roles.

Duplication or overlap in prescribing roles has not materialised. For example, within the specialty of rheumatology, doctors, nurses, podiatrists and physiotherapists already engage in prescribing activities, without confusion over role boundaries or responsibilities. Supplementary prescribing in particular also appears to be geared towards ensuring an effective alternative to doctor prescribing in key, defined areas of practice, not as an addition to it. Alarmist concerns that extended prescribing will translate directly into excessive prescribing have no basis in fact.

Above all, it is now clear that a wide variety of AHPs are successfully undertaking new and evolving roles across the spectrum of prescribing. Each profession employs subtly different prescribing activities, tailored to particular needs within specific clinical contexts. Given the opportunity to engage fully with independent prescribing, these discrete prescribing patterns would undoubtedly emerge with greater clarity. Most AHP professions possess a range of specialist areas of practice, recognised in some way as distinct from generalist practice, with unique prescribing requirements. Current AHP prescribing activity reflects the specific skills, experience and expertise of the practitioners concerned. In the context of prescribing, therefore, AHP practitioners are not merely substitute physicians. Rather, AHP prescribing is part of an ongoing reshaping of the healthcare workforce which is increasingly utilising the expertise and skill of the AHPs. In reality, many of the AHPs have been accustomed to accessing and administering restricted medicines for many years, and the advent of supplementary or independent prescribing will simply enable a fuller expression of the range of skills and expertise of these groups within their fields of competence.

An appreciation of the clinical context is critical to any understanding of the breadth of AHP prescribing. For example, specialist podiatric surgeons require access to a distinctive range of specific medicines, very different than that required by generalist podiatrists. Effective bone penetration is a required property of any anti-biotic used in the management of bone infections, a rare but serious complication in foot surgery. Thus, access to, and administration of, clinically effective doses of clindamycin, or perhaps sodium fusidate, are essential components of a podiatric surgeon's armamentarium, yet these agents are not ever likely to be sought by general podiatric practitioners. Similarly, the required mode of administration of a medicine may vary, according to the specific circumstances. For example, in cases of deep post-operative infection, a podiatric surgeon may choose to temporarily implant gentamicin-impregnated acrylic beads into a surgical wound, to be replaced with other relevant therapies thereafter. Similar decisions would probably be made by orthopaedic surgeons faced with the same dilemma. Yet, until podiatric surgeons can independently prescribe these agents as required, the situation will remain unnecessarily problematic, placing needless demands on physician's time and delaying essential patient care.

As mentioned earlier, extended scope physiotherapists commonly possess specialist skills in the parenteral administration of certain medicines. They are often experienced in their use, yet remain unable to legally administer the necessary medicines without a physician's patient specific direction (or PGD in the NHS). If the move towards greater AHP prescribing is to succeed, instances such as these will need to be addressed. By affording ESPs the legal freedom to administer required medicines, the advantages for patients, AHPs and physicians alike will be clear to see. Reluctance on the part of the medical profession to unequivocally support extended AHP prescribing has stemmed from a fear of over-prescribing, the possibility of increased risks of anti-biotic resistance, and the creation of a cadre of inadequately trained, non-medical prescribers. Despite all evidence to the contrary, it is likely that the medical profession will continue to exhibit a certain aversion to independent prescribing by non-medically qualified professionals, as it continues to resist a further, progressive erosion in medical autonomy (DoH, 2007c; Gabe *et al.*, 1994). Nevertheless, providing the prevailing climate in government policy remains focused on ensuring an adaptive, flexible healthcare workforce, it is likely that AHP independent prescribing will, in due course, become an accepted, normative practice. No doubt much will depend on the success, or otherwise, of pharmacy and nurse independent prescribing.

REFERENCES

Abbott, A. (1988) *The System of Professions – An Essay on the Division of Expert Labour.* Chicago: University of Chicago Press.

Adonis, A. (1993) *Parliament Today.* Manchester, UK: University of Manchester Press.

Allarton, A. (2006) Cited in: Is education fit for purpose? *News and Events, Frontline*, 15 November 2006, http://www.csp.org.uk/director/newsandevents/frontline/archiveissues (accessed on 11 April 2007).

Blake, A. (2005) A post-operative comparison of nail avulsion using phenol and cryotherapy. *British Journal of Podiatry*, **8**, 128–32.

BMJ (1967a) Editorial: control of drugs. *British Medical Journal*, 16 September, pp. 689–90.

BMJ (1967b) Proposed legislation on drugs. *British Medical Journal*, 16 September, p. 734.

Borthwick, A. M. (1997) A Study of the Professionalisation Strategies of British Podiatry 1960–1997. Unpublished Ph.D. thesis, University of Salford.

Borthwick, A. M. (2000) Challenging medicine: the case of podiatric surgery. *Work, Employment and Society (Notes and Issues)*, **14**(2), 369–383.

Borthwick, A. M. (2001a) Drug prescribing in podiatry: radicalism or tokenism? *British Journal of Podiatry*, **4**, 56–64.

Borthwick, A. M. (2001b) Predicting the impact of new prescribing rights. *guest editorial. The Diabetic Foot*, **4**(1), 4–8.

Borthwick, A. M. (2002) Attaining prescribing rights: miracle or mirage? editorial. *Podiatry Now*, **5**, 158.

Borthwick, A. M. (2003) Prescribing rights for the allied health professions: temporary lull or quiet abandonment? *Podium*, **1**(4), 4–6.

Borthwick, A. M. (2004) The politics of allied health prescribing: reflections on a new discourse, editorial. *British Journal of Podiatry*, **7**, 31.

Borthwick, A. M. (2005) 'In the beginning': local anaesthesia and the Croydon Postgraduate Group. *British Journal of Podiatry*, **8**, 87–94.

Borthwick, A. M. & Nancarrow, S. (2005) Promoting health: the role of the specialist podiatrist. In: Scriven, A. (ed), *Health Promoting Practice – The Contribution of Nurses and Allied Health Professionals*. Basingstoke, UK: Palgrave Macmillan.

Bowen, C. (2003) Podiatric Rheumatic Care Association. *Podiatry Now*, **6**(6), 18.

Bradlow, J. & Coulter, A. (1993) Effect of fundholding and indicative prescribing scheme on general practitioners' prescribing costs. *British Medical Journal*, **307**, 1186–9.

Cameron, A. & Masterson, A. (2003) Reconfiguring the clinical workforce. In: Davies, C. (ed), *The Future Health Workforce*. Basingstoke, UK: Palgrave Macmillan.

The Chiropodist (1980) State registered chiropodists: local analgesia. *The Chiropodist*, **35**, 279.

CoR (1996) *Role Development in Radiography*. London: College of Radiographers.

CoR (2001) *Prescribing by Radiographers: A Vision Paper*. London: College of Radiographers.

CoR (2007) *Course of Study for the Certification of Competence in Administering Intravenous Injections*. London: College of Radiographers.

CSP (1999) *A Clinical Guideline for the Use of Injection Therapy by Physical Therapists*. London: Chartered Society of Physiotherapists.

CSP (2003) *Prescribing Rights for Physiotherapists*. PA 58. London: Chartered Society of Physiotherapists.

CSP (2005) *Prescribing Rights for Physiotherapists; An Update*. Chartered Society of Physiotherapists. London: CSP.

Cumming, S., Stewart, S., Harborne, D., Smith, J., Broom, H., Abbott, A. & Barton A. (2005) A randomised controlled trial of phenol and sodium hydroxide in nail surgery. *British Journal of Podiatry*, **8**, 123–7.

Department of Health (1994) *Feet First – Report of the Joint Department of Health and NHS Chiropody Task Force*. Department of Health 1085, 16M, 9/94. London: Department of Health.

Department of Health (1999) *Final Report of the Review of Prescribing, Supply and Administration of Medicines (Crown Report)*. London: Department of Health.

Department of Health (2000a) *Patient Group Directions – Guidance on Group Directions*. Health Service Circular, HSC2000/026 (England only). London: Department of Health.

Department of Health (2000b) *Patient Group Directions*. Health Service Circular, NHS HDL (2001)7 (Scotland only). London: Department of Health.

Department of Health (2000c) *Patient Group Directions*. Health Service Circular, WHC2000/16 (Wales only). London: Department of Health.

Department of Health (2001) *The NHS Plan – A Plan for Investment, a Plan for Reform*. London: Department of Health.

Department of Health (2005) *Supplementary Prescribing by Nurses, Pharmacists, Chiropodists/ Podiatrists, Physiotherapists and Radiographers within the NHS in England*. London: Department of Health.

Department of Health (2007a) *Commissioning Toolkit for Community Based Eye Services*. London: Department of Health.

Department of Health (2007b) Patient Group Directions, http://www.dh.gov.uk/en/ Policyandguidance/ Emergencyplanning/DH_4069610 (accessed 23 April 2007).

Department of Health (2007c) *Trust, Assurance and Safety – The Regulation of Health Professionals in the 21st Century*. London: Department of Health.

Dickson, D. J. (1996) What do general practitioners expect from rheumatology clinics? *British Journal of Rheumatology*, **35**, 920.

Evans, R. (2004) CEO Society of Radiographers, cited in Radiographers to receive prescription rights. *Synergy News*, June issue, p. 6.

Fournier, V. (2000) Boundary work and the (un)making of the professions. In: Malin, N. (ed), *Professionalism, Boundaries and the Workplace*. London: Routledge.

Francis, G. & Hogg, D. (2006) Radiographer prescribing: enhancing seamless care in oncology. *Radiography*, **12**, 3–5.

Freeman, C. (2006) Professional Officer, Society and College of Radiographers, cited in Work on radiographer prescribing gathers pace. *Synergy News*, June issue, p. 7.

Freidson, E. (1970a) *Professional Dominance – The Social Structure of Medical Care*. New York: Atherton Press.

Freidson, E. (1970b) *Profession of Medicine – A Study of the Sociology of Applied Knowledge*. Chicago: University of Chicago Press.

Freidson, E. (1994) *Professionalism Reborn – Theory, Prophecy and Policy*. Cambridge, UK: Polity Press.

Freidson, E. (2001) *Professionalism: The Third Logic*. Oxford, UK: Oxford University Press.

Frontline (2004) CSP continues to push for prescribing rights for physio. London: CSP, 15 September 2004, http://www.csp.org.uk/director/newsandevents/frontline/archiveissues.cfm.

Gabe, J. Kelleher, D. & Williams, G. (1994) *Challenging Medicine*. London: Routledge.

Ham, C. (1994) *Management and Competition in the New NHS*. Oxford, UK: Radcliffe Medical Press.

Ham, C. (2002) *Health Policy in Britain*, 5th edn. Basingstoke, UK: Palgrave Macmillan.

Health Professions Council (2007) Register of Approved Course-Supplementary Prescribing, http://www.hpc-uk.org/aboutregistration/educationandtraining/approvedcourses_sp/ (accessed on 28 May 2007).

Health and Social Care Act (2001) Part 5, Clause 68. The Stationery Office: London, 2001.

Hogg, P., Francis, G., Hogg, D., Mountain, V., Pitt, A., Sherrington, S. & Freeman C. (2007) Prescription, supply and administration of medicines in radiography: current position and future directions. *Synergy News*, December 2007, 27–31.

Hogg, D. & Hogg, P. (2003) Guest editorial, Radiographer prescribing: lessons to be learnt from the community nursing experience. *Radiography*, **9**, 263–5.

Hogg, P. & Hogg, D. (2006) Prescription, supply and administration of drugs in diagnosis and therapy. *Synergy News*, March issue, pp. 4–8.

JBPM (1994) Forging ahead with prescription only medicines. *Journal of British Podiatric Medicine*, **49**(1), 2.

Kerr, D. & Richardson, T. (2000) The diabetic foot at the crossroads: vanguard or oblivion? *The Diabetic Foot*, **3**, 70–1.

Kirkbride, P. & Craig, A. (2006) 3SI or how to reduce radiotherapy waiting times. *Synergy News*, April issue, pp. 12–14.

Larkin, G. V. (1979) Medical dominance and control: radiographers in the division of labour. *Sociological Review*, **26**, 843–58.

Larkin, G. V. (1980) Professionalism, dentistry and public health. *Social Science and Medicine*, **14a**, 223–9.

Larkin, G. V. (1981) Professional autonomy and the ophthalmic optician. *Sociology of Health and Illness*, **3**(1), 15–30.

Larkin, G. V. (1983) *Occupational Monopoly and Medicine*. London: Tavistock.

Larkin, G. V. (1988) Medical dominance in Britain – image and historical reality. *Millbank Quarterly* **66**(Suppl 3), 117–32.

Larkin, G. V. (1993) Continuity in change: medical dominance in the United Kingdom. In: Hafferty, F. & McKinlay, J. (eds), *The Changing Medical Profession: An International Perspective*. Oxford, UK: Oxford University Press.

Larkin, G. V. (1995) State control and the health professions in the United Kingdom: historical perspectives. In: Johnson, T., Larkin, G. & Saks, M. (eds), *Health Professions and the State in Europe*. London: Routledge.

Lawrenson, J. G. (2005) Recent changes in the use and supply of medicines by optometrists. *Optometry Today*, 3 June, pp. 28–32.

Lawrenson, J. G. (2007) Academic Committee and Research Sub-Committee, College of Optometrists, telephone interview, 19 April 2007.

Limb, M. (2005) Blurring boundaries. *Frontline, News and Events*, 1 September 2005, http://www.csp.org.uk/director/newsandevents/frontline/archiveissues (accessed 11 April 2007).

Limb, M. (2006) Supplementary question. *Frontline, News and Events*, 16 August 2006a, http://www.csp.org.uk/director/newsandevents/frontline/archiveissues (accessed 11 April 2007).

Malin, N., Wilmot, S. & Manthorpe, J. (2002) *Key Concepts and Debates in Health and Social Policy*. Maidenhead, UK: Open University Press.

McCartney, W., Tyrer, S., Brazier, M. & Prayle, D. (1999) Nurse prescribing: radicalism or tokenism? *Journal of Advanced Nursing*, **29**, 348–54.

McInnes, A. (2002) Are podiatrists qualified for the job? *The Diabetic Foot*, **5**, 62–7.

Medicines Act (1968) London: The Stationery Office.

MHRA (2003) *Sale, Supply and Administration of Medicines by Allied Health Professionals under Patient Group Directions*, MLX294. London: Medicines and Helthcare Products Regulatory Agency.

MHRA (2004) *Proposals for the Amendments to the Range of Medicines Which Can Be Sold, Supplied or Administered by Optometrists*, MLX306. London: Medicines and Healthare Products Regulatory Agency.

MHRA (2006) *Medicines for Human Use (Administration and Sale or Supply)* (Miscellaneous Amendments) Order 2006, Statutory Instrument 2006 No. 2807. London: The Stationery Office.

Needle, J., Lawrenson, J. G. & Petchley, R. (2007) *Scope of Therapeutic Practice: A Survey of UK Optometrists: A Report Prepared for the College of Optometrists*. London: City University London.

The Opticians Act (1958), London: HMSO.

Oxlade, L. (2006) Is education fit for practice? *Frontline News and Events*, 1 November 2006, http://www.csp.org.uk/director/newsandevents/frontline/archiveissues (accessed 11 April 2007).

Robinson, P. (2004) Cited in CSP continues to push for prescribing rights for physios. *Frontline, News and Events*, 15 September 2004, http://www.csp.org.uk/director/newsandevents/frontline/archiveissues (accessed 11 April 2007).

SCoR (2002) *Submission Document in Response to Review of Prescribing, Supply and Administration of Medicines (Crown II) Final Report*. March 1999 (including appendices A and B). London: Society and College of Radiographers.

SCP (2004) Minutes of meeting of medicines committee. London: Society of Chiropodists and Podiatrists, 5 February.

SCP (2006a) *Podiatry Medicines Access and Supply Updated Pharmacology Syllabus*. London: Society of Chiropodists & Podiatrists.

SCP (2006b), Minutes of meeting of medicines committee. London: Society of Chiropodists and Podiatrists, 19 January.

SCP (2006c) Minutes of meeting of medicines committee. London: Society of Chiropodists and Podiatrists, 6 September.

SCP (2007) Minutes of meeting of medicines committee. London: Society of Chiropodists and Podiatrists, 21 February.

Shepherd, J. (2000) Changes in roles and responsibilities: a personal view. *Synergy News*, March issue, p. 20.

Synergy News (2003) First therapy consultant says role is a major advance. *Synergy News*, October issue, p. 3.

Synergy News (2004) Radiographers to receive prescription rights. *Synergy News*, June issue, p. 6.

Synergy News (2006a) Radiographer prescribing of medicines. *Synergy News*, November issue, p. 11.

Synergy News (2006b) Trainee therapy consultant looks forward to a successful career. *Synergy News*, February issue, p. 9.

Taylor, R. S. (1999) Partnerships or power struggles? The crown review of prescribing. *British Journal of General Practice*, **49**, 340–1.

Timmons, S. & Tanner, J. (2004) A disputed occupational boundary: operating theatre nurses and operating department practitioners. *Sociology of Health and Illness*, **26**, 645–66.

Titcomb, L. C. & Lawrenson, J. G. (2006) Recent changes in medicines legislation that affect optometrists. *Optometry in Practice*, **7**, 23–34.

Webster, C. (2002) The National Health Service: A Political History, 2nd edn. Oxford, UK: Oxford University Press.

Young, M. (2002) When Is a Diabetic Specialist Not a DSP? *The Diabetic Foot*, **5**(2), 5–7.

Young, M. (2003) Generalists, specialists and super-specialists. *The Diabetic Foot*, **6**(1), 6.

Conclusions

Peter Nolan and Eleanor Bradley

Non-medical prescribing was one of many innovations introduced into health care at the beginning of the twenty-first century. Nurses were the first group to be involved, with other professional groups subsequently acquiring prescribing rights. The reform of the public sector was a cornerstone of the Labour Government manifesto which sought to make health services accountable, flexible and accessible to all at the point of need (Department of Health [DoH], 2006b). The scaffolding upon which the modernisation of the National Health Service (NHS) has been constructed during the last decade has been the creation of new structures and roles, increased spending and greater emphasis on the measurement of outcomes. The NHS is a diverse organisation, embracing a myriad of disciplines, each with its own history, philosophy and practices. A consequence of this diversity is that even small changes can be problematic. Given the extent of the changes introduced over the last decade, future analysts of healthcare will probably claim that much of the funding allocated during this time was spent on the *introduction* of change rather than the *delivery of care*. This is not necessarily inappropriate because good-quality care requires robust systems to underpin and support it as well as methods of monitoring and measuring effectiveness.

The aim of this book was to focus on one aspect of the modernisation agenda, namely, non-medical prescribing. By examining the experiences of those involved, including professional colleagues and service users, the authors set out to reach some conclusions about the impact of non-medical prescribing as well as critique the process of change in a modern complex healthcare system. Preceding chapters have demonstrated that, at the initiation of non-medical prescribing, there was considerable agreement among professionals about its merits and about how the new role should be introduced and supported, but there were also differences of opinion. There were differences not only within and between professional groups but also in the vision as specified by health policies and the experience of practitioners on the ground. This may not be surprising, given that policy documents tend to paint 'the big picture', whereas service providers are limited as to what they can do by their environment and remit. Before attempting to draw conclusions from what has been presented in previous chapters, it is important to emphasise that the book has examined the experiences of those who were in the *vanguard* of the non-medical prescribing initiative and to point out that this initiative is still in its infancy and is developing almost day by day. Currently, it holds a marginal position in non-medical professions, and it will take some time for it to be integrated and accepted as a mainstream activity in all services. It is possible that the first cohorts of non-medical prescribers will prove to be different from those now following on; they may be more confident, more highly motivated and have stronger beliefs in the value of what they are doing. They may also be people who under-report problems or exaggerate the benefits of a particular innovation when they are involved in it.

It must be acknowledged that it is not possible to say to what extent the views presented in this book would be representative of those of personnel and services across the UK. Nonetheless, important issues have been raised about change in general in the NHS and about non-medical prescribing in particular. Nationwide, the up-take of non-medical prescribing has been patchy, with some Trusts and individuals embracing it enthusiastically and others giving it a low priority. With a plethora of new roles being introduced simultaneously, some personnel who opted to train as non-medical prescribers may move to other roles in which prescribing is not required. Just as there is attrition at junior staff level, especially in nursing, attrition is also problematic at more senior levels. Staff may be attracted to new posts in universities, in clinical governance, clinical audit, operational services and human resources, thus depriving the clinical arena of their expertise and experience. The irony may be that, to deliver the modernisation programme, personnel with excellent clinical credentials are diverted into managerial roles.

The contribution of this book to understanding the NHS today, and the process of change within it, is to provide a glimpse of how those involved in an innovation that was a radical departure from traditional NHS culture perceived and responded to it. The number of individuals and professional groups involved in non-medical prescribing is slowly increasing but has not escalated at the rate expected by the DoH. Many of those who elected to become prescribers encountered barriers which exposed deeply entrenched managerial and professional attitudes prevalent within healthcare as well as the ingrained prejudices of certain individuals. The chapters of this book reveal the generally conservative nature of the health service, and the – occasionally extreme – caution with which people view and implement change. Although non-medical prescribing had been discussed in the UK for nearly two decades before being rolled out to professionals across healthcare services, many medical staff appeared to be oblivious or indifferent to it and were taken by surprise when it finally arrived. As Campbell observes in Chapter 2, it was late in the day before some doctors realised that non-medical prescribing signalled the colonisation of territory which had traditionally been their preserve by disciplines with very different attitudes from theirs to healthcare and prescribing. On the other hand, as Borthwick argues in Chapter 7, non-medical prescribing might also signal the medicalisation of non-medical groups and an even wider acceptance that pharmacological treatments are the dominant intervention in healthcare. After all, it is doctors who are expected to mentor non-medical prescribers during and after their training.

It is evident that a radical change in the role of one professional group can have profound implications for other groups, yet policy makers appear to have underestimated the tensions that result when challenging policies are introduced in haste. Role re-alignment has the potential to disrupt multi-disciplinary working, unless people are able to manage change within themselves, and also in those around them.

The historical perspective presented in Chapter 1 demonstrates that change has been an integral part of healthcare throughout the decades and prescribing practices have always been characterised by rituals and protocols. Following in the footsteps of ancient healers, doctors gradually extended their remit so that they defined the aetiology of diseases, they determined what counted as illness, they prescribed treatments for illnesses and, most importantly, they acted as gatekeepers to services provided by others. It has perhaps always been true that, given the power and influence of the medical profession, many patients have taken prescribed drugs, not because they have found them useful but in order to please their doctors (Kinnersley *et al.*, 1999)!

By the end of the twentieth century, the growth of medical practice, coupled with the demands of the public for better health and better healthcare, were putting the NHS under considerable strain. However generously funded, the healthcare system could not afford to provide services at the rate at which they were being consumed and alternatives had to be found. Given that the population was better informed than previous generations and had access to a wider range of health-promoting consumables and facilities, it seemed reasonable to encourage people to take responsibility for their own health. The rise of 'healthism' sees a return to a medieval concept of holistic health care which incorporates health promotion, attention to diet and exercise, and natural treatments, such as herbal medicines that can be bought from health food shops. Naidoo and Wills (2000) point to the growing market in complementary and alternative therapies as evidence that increasing numbers of people, and especially those who have conditions that have not been successfully treated, are dissatisfied with invasive, impersonal medicine.

Changes in how members of the general public perceive their health, and the health services they want, will inevitably affect what professionals do in the future and the types of care they provide. Whereas doctors have always been clear about their role, other professional groups, especially nurses, have been less so. The arrival of new nursing roles (see Chapter 2) could lead to a fragmentation of nursing rather than greater unification. Health professionals allied to medicine could see their roles strengthened and more clearly defined. Some prescribing professionals may be tempted to adopt a more medical orientation to their work, losing the outlook of their 'native' profession and seeing themselves as 'mini-doctors'. This poses some challenging questions which are unlikely to be answered without a critical mass of prescribers within each profession. If non-medical prescribing does relieve the burden on doctors, what will the role of the doctor look like? What new responsibilities will doctors take on to demonstrate that they are having a significant impact on the health of the nation? What aspects of the doctors previous roles will non-medical prescribers jettison as they assume greater responsibility for the management of medicines? There is a real danger that leaving these questions unresolved will result in some personnel becoming overloaded, burned out and eventually abandoning their prescribing role.

The authors who have contributed to this book can see the emphasis in pre-scribing shifting away slowly from the treatment of illness, or the mere alleviation of symptoms, towards the promotion and maintenance of health. Resources are to be concentrated on vulnerable groups in the population and to assist those with severe and enduring disabilities to live more fulfilled lives. Epidemiological studies show that despite the best efforts of policy makers and service commis-sioners, considerable health inequalities are still apparent across the nation. Does non-medical prescribing have a role in addressing these inequalities? Will non-medical prescribing assist the 'hard-to-reach' groups? Will it encourage 'entrepreneurialism' so that professionals develop innovative services such as drop-in centres, well-person clinics, children's centres and community-based clinics? Will a 'top-down' approach to the modernisation of health services be replaced by 'bottom-up' approaches that respond to what people want? The non-medical prescribers whose views are presented in this book appear keen to provide services that are user centred and empowering. They seem to favour the emerging paradigm which proposes that taking responsibility for one's health enhances personal autonomy and which views traditional approaches to the management of illness as disabling.

Both healthcare personnel and service users live in constantly changing, com-plex worlds and become preoccupied trying to make sense of them. Improve-ment, as personnel see it, means giving service users more time, seeing problems from the perspective of the person as well as the diagnostician, and providing tai-lored advice and information. While all non-medical prescribers were anxious about their inability to diagnose, and some their limited knowledge of pharma-cology, they nonetheless contended that good prescribing is grounded in human relations and not solely in medical sciences. Prescribers needed to recognise that most illnesses are self-limiting and that the quality of the relationship between the carer and the cared allows for insight into when medicines are required and when they are not. Non-medical prescribers did not underestimate the power of the body and mind to heal themselves, and they understood that people's knowledge and interpretation of their conditions affect their recovery. Indeed, it has been proposed that the meaning attributed by a person to his or her illness and health can affect the way in which medications work on their physiology and psychology (Moerman, 2002).

Non-medical prescribers highlighted the importance of the consultation which may lead to medicines being prescribed. Services users have described not being listened to, not being given information and not having the chance to explore alternatives to medicines as infuriating when consulting health professionals (Lundkvist *et al.*, 2002). The quality of the relationship between prescriber and client is an essential part of the prescribing process. Both participants bring to it their own expectations, their own perceptions of illness and treatment, their own interpretation of what the evidence says and their own beliefs about what constitutes optimum health. Physical, psychological, social and spiritual definitions of health overlap with implications for the individual's well-being. Hypotheses are stated and tested, and personal and cultural beliefs and values are challenged. The consultation may be stressful and requires a high degree of trust on the part of both participants. The service user has to decide whether the prescriber can be trusted with his or her welfare and whether adopting the recommended course of action will result in improved health. Equally, judgements are made by the prescriber as to whether the client and members of his or her family will engage with the treatment plan. Chapter 5 describes the importance of managing the prescribing relationship successfully. Indeed, the existence of a trusting and open relationship between clinicians and patients can lead to outcomes which are far more favourable to both parties.

Although this book reveals similarities in the experiences of allied health professionals (AHPs) and nurse prescribers on their journeys towards prescriptive authority, there are also key differences. In particular, there appears to be less concern among AHPs that prescribing will fundamentally alter the way in which they are seen by service users and multi-disciplinary team members. Allied health professionals operate in clearly defined areas, and have instantly recognisable skills (despite being grouped together as AHPs). It is acknowledged that they have very specific expertise within highly specialised areas of practice and that their work is quite different from the 'generalist' practice of most nurses. Unlike AHPs, nurses faced a major challenge in fitting prescribing into their current roles, explaining it to multi-disciplinary team members and working as prescribers alongside medical colleagues.

The prescribing role has huge potential to develop the practice of AHPs, particularly their ability to complete an episode of care. Many have been prescribing 'informally' for years but, like nurse prescribers, may face resistance from medical colleagues when they become formally qualified as prescribers. They will need to explain their remit clearly and negotiate skilfully to establish their new role within the multi-disciplinary team.

To develop the non-medical prescribing initiative in the future, it is vital that lessons are learnt from experiences during early implementation. This book has highlighted that the following areas are key in establishing the effectiveness of non-medical prescribing.

Benefits for service users

It is ultimately service users who will decide on the success or otherwise of non-medical prescribing. Benefits, if there are any, will only become apparent following thorough evaluation of developing services. It is reassuring that the accounts of service users reported in Chapter 5 were highly supportive. However, the fact that they were service users identified by the new non-medical prescribers themselves may mean that they are not typical of service users more generally. What the service users valued most, as identified in other studies, was primarily having more time with a helpful and friendly professional. More time permitted health carers to get closer to individuals so that service users could learn more about their condition, gain a better understanding of their medicines and thereby manage them more effectively. More time for questioning enabled service users to retain more of what was said to them and encouraged them to assume greater responsibility for their own health care. Research in health education (Ladenpera & Kyngas, 2000) has shown that informing and educating services users about their condition, offering a range of treatments and encouraging them to believe that they will recover, enhances the likelihood that their condition will improve. Genuine, therapeutic relationships also result in fewer drug errors and drug wastage.

There are a number of key aspects to prescribing relationships that are appreciated by service users:
- Having sufficient time to talk about their problems
- Contact with a clinician who is knowledgeable, experienced and sympathetic
- Being listened to, believed and understood
- Being able to state their beliefs about illness and health
- Having their strengths identified and valued
- Being able to discuss treatments, alternatives and side effects
- Having their lifestyle and commitments taken into account
- Being given choice of interventions that improve health rather than merely address symptoms
- Ultimately, being involved in *all aspects* of the consultation

Prescribing: pre-requisite skills and training

There is a temptation during periods of transition in healthcare for personnel to become overly enthusiastic about new developments and to 'jump on the bandwagon'. However, fears that non-medical prescribing might unleash a wave of prescribing have proved unfounded, suggesting that there is a stronger degree of self-regulation being exercised by those choosing to become prescribers than was thought might be the case.

Non-medical prescribing is a key component of government healthcare policy, and the extent to which it will develop in the future will depend largely on how confident, competent and safe the personnel selected to become prescribers prove themselves to be. An assessment of those selected to become prescribers must be carried out from many perspectives, and practice requirements must be constantly borne in mind. It is preferable that prescribers should have detailed understanding of the physiological and pharmacological effects of medicines and of their associated complications. Factors such as age, training, skills, disposition and ambition all require consideration, and different posts require different combinations of key qualities. Ultimately, new roles are created by post holders and organisations working in partnership. This makes it imperative that prescribers from all disciplines are clear about their unique contribution to care and resist the temptation of assuming low-level medical roles. The more complex the care required by patients, the more necessity there is for health professionals to collaborate. While initial preparation for prescribing may ideally be differentiated according to discipline, trusts should adopt a collaborative approach to continued professional development (CPD). This will facilitate consistency, enable prescribers to appreciate the breadth of knowledge and expertise within their organisation, and enhance understanding of different approaches to treatment and care. The assessment of competence in prescribers who qualified prior to the new NMC standards should be revisited, along with availability of and access to CPD. Including nurse prescribing in the Key Skills Framework (KSF) requires greater commitment from organisations. Regular audits of prescribing activity across the range of settings within which nurse prescribers are working are vital.

The decision to become a prescriber is a weighty one. Some may see it primarily as a career opportunity or a chance to work more autonomously; the majority, however, see it as a means to improve services and assist service users, especially those with long-term conditions. The evidence from previous chapters indicates that those who chose to train at the start of the non-medical prescribing initiative had extensive experience, were confident within their professional roles, felt informed about pharmacological interventions and were highly motivated to provide better services. This was important because they needed to be able to command the respect of their peers and of other professionals as well as to negotiate with complex organisations. It was also important that as they took on prescribing, they were able to let go of other work to avoid burnout.

It was evident that not all pharmacists or nurses were clear about what prescribing training consisted of or what their future prescribing roles would entail.

They were committing to an ideal rather than to a reality, because few of them at that stage had witnessed other non-medical prescribers in practice. It would appear now that the following characteristics and abilities are important in professionals contemplating non-medical prescribing:

- Security within their profession
- Access to regular, high-quality supervision
- Sound leadership skills
- Understanding of the physiological and pharmacological effects of medicines
- Vision as to how non-medical prescribing can improve services for those with disabling and long-term conditions
- Skills in negotiation and discussion
- Skills in challenging and confronting
- Innovation
- Ability to transfer skills from one role to another
- Ability to integrate prescribing into their work
- Preparedness to integrate assessment, information giving and health-promotion activities into their work with service users

Current issues in prescribing training

Training programmes are useful for conveying knowledge and cognitive skills, but may be less effective in conferring competence and confidence. Many of the nurses whose voices are heard in Chapters 4, 5 and 6 found that prescribing training made them very anxious and felt that they had not been fully supported to manage their fears. In addition to knowledge, it is important to appreciate that students need assistance to become more confident when applying training. Furthermore, increased confidence would render them more likely to experience enhanced job satisfaction. Hence, the challenge to education providers, in addition to instilling good practice in students, is also to assist them with acquiring high levels of self-esteem, skills in self-management and the foresight to be self-directed.

Sending personnel on courses has proved disappointing in some areas of healthcare because the climate in which they are expected to implement what they have learned is resistant to change (Fadden, 1997; Tarrier et al., 1998). In Chapter 2, it was reported that professionals taking one of the first prescribing courses were bitterly disappointed by the limitations placed on their prescribing practice post-qualification. Courses may raise expectations, but it is ultimately the quality and flexibility of the working environment that determine the extent to which training can be implemented. In the instance cited above, the course participants protested and were instrumental in changing the prescribing course for the better.

The following are important issues to bear in mind in selecting personnel for non-medical prescribing courses:

- To identify personnel with experience and understanding of a range of treatments in addition to pharmacological interventions
- To identify students who are self-motivated and self-directed
- To recognise those who can learn from and in practice

In addition, it is important that those coming forward for training should have identified, or be helped to identify, role models and mentors; that lecturers should be competent in the skills they are attempting to convey; and that higher education institutions (HEIs) collaborate with healthcare organisations to ensure that there are ample opportunities for students to test in practice what has been learned in the classroom.

The inclusion of nurses from a range of specialties on the prescribing course was viewed positively by participants, despite representing a significant challenge to lecturers. Training courses are encouraged to be multi-disciplinary as a means of stimulating discussion, promoting team working and assisting the implementation of skills in practice. Universities providing non-medical prescribing courses should be encouraged to consider the use of teachers from different sectors in the training course, including the independent and voluntary sectors, to enable trainees to fully consider the potential for prescribing, share experiences, challenge current prescribing practices and think about innovation in their workplaces.

It would seem clear from this book that candidates for non-medical prescribing training need to be experienced nurses, with excellent communication skills, who are clear that they will have a role in their team as a prescriber, and who are committed to prescribing. Beyond the selection issue are wider considerations to do with the workforce. The number of non-medical prescribers per team requires careful thought. Questions remain unanswered as to whether a sole prescriber can function well within a team, and whether this provides equity of access for all service users. If a team decides to have just one nurse prescriber, does this deny other nurses equality of opportunity to train as prescribers?

This book has suggested that the preparation of nurses as non-medical prescribers may be lacking because it has focused predominantly on imparting *knowledge*, rather than on the *processes* of prescribing. This has led to difficulties for non-medical prescribers, particularly those working either in isolation, without ready sources of support of guidance, or in teams that are not supportive of prescribing. Providers of education also need to consider revising prescribing programmes in light of the needs of *all* healthcare staff to avoid the need to 'upgrade' every time a new statutory instrument is put in place. Pre-registration training programmes for AHPs and nurses must prepare professionals for future extended roles and, in the case of nurses, provide increased education in pharmacology, thus ensuring nurses a smooth transition to postgraduate prescribing courses.

Non-medical prescribers and doctors

It cannot be over-stated that empowering one group and extending its role can threaten another. To date, little attention has been given to the impact of non-medical prescribing on the medical profession despite the fact that without the assistance of doctors, it stands little chance of being implemented. Doctors have generally been trained to assume responsibility for every service user and for all aspects of the service in which they are working. Senior medical staff are accustomed to shouldering a considerable burden of responsibility and may be suspicious of those seeking to take some of that burden from them. This book has suggested that doctors may be fearful of nurses and AHPs attempting to become, as they see it, 'mini-doctors'. Where nurse prescribers are members of the multi-disciplinary team, there is evidence that doctors have started to renegotiate their roles, sometimes as 'medical managers', to address their concerns about nurses assuming total responsibility for patients. They argue that prescribing necessitates assessment and diagnostic skills and that these are not covered in detail either during pre-registration or prescribing training.

It may be helpful for non-medical prescribers to consider that their medical colleagues:

- Have resisted, to varying degrees, attempts to regulate their profession and their practice
- Attend the meetings of other professional colleagues infrequently
- Guard their professional boundaries and resist challenges to their power and position
- Have traditionally worked more closely with nurses than with any other group, but the balance of power within that collaboration has been unequal

Gaining the respect and confidence of medical staff is vital for non-medical prescribers who need to make clear what it is they can offer to doctors. Advice should be given sensitively, offers made to participate in clinical consultations, and evidence provided that the contribution of non-medical prescribers is a valid one.

A supportive team, with a clear understanding of the role of the non-medical prescriber, can help shape the new role realistically and ensure that those who occupy it practise safely. The issue of safety is of prime importance and is especially acute for non-medical prescribers working in isolation for long periods. It is increasingly the case that not all teams are based at the same location, and this can be problematic in terms of collaboration and joined-up working. Since the Shipman Enquiry (2004), best practice is defined as that which is carried out by a team, members of which work closely together, support each other and are supervised and appraised.

This book makes clear that despite initial anxieties, and regardless of their eventual prescribing activity, the first cohorts of nurse and AHP prescribers have derived a number of personal and professional benefits from undertaking prescribing training. These include improved knowledge, enhanced self-esteem and increased job satisfaction. Provided that organisational and team support is available, there is every reason to be confident that the non-medical prescribing initiative will reap rich rewards for both health professionals and service users. In the UK, non-medical prescribing has been a major innovation. There is no doubt that it has already made a significant contribution to the lives of some service users. Only time can reveal whether that contribution will have a measurable effect on the health of the nation.

REFERENCES

Corrigan, P. W. & McCracken, S. G. (1995b) Re-focusing the training of psychiatric rehabilitation staff. *Psychiatric Services*, **46**, 1172–7.

Department of Health (2006b) *Our Health, Our Care, Our Say: A New Direction for Community Services*. London: HMSO.

Fadden, G. (1997) Implementation of family interventions in routine clinical practice following staff programmes: a major cause for concern. *Journal of Mental Health*, **6**, 599–12.

Kavanagh, D. J., Piatkowska, O., Clark, D., O'Harroran, P. *et al.* (1993) Application of cognitive behavioural family intervention for schizophrenia in multidisciplinary teams: what can the matter be? *Australian Psychologist*, **28**, 181–8.

Kinnersley, P., Stott, N., Peters, T. J. & Harvey, I. (1999) The patient-centeredness of consultations and outcomes in primary care. *British Journal of General Practice*, **49**, 711–16.

Ladenpera, T. & Kyngas, H. (2000) Compliance and its evaluation in patients with hypertension. *Journal of Clinical Nursing*, **9**, 826–33.

Lundkvist, J., Akerlind, I., Borgquist, L. & Molstad, S. (2002) The more time spent on listening, the less time spent on prescribing antibiotics in general practice. *Family Practice*, **19**, 638–40.

Moerman, D. (2002) *Meaning, Medicine and the 'Placebo Effect'*. Cambridge, UK: Cambridge University Press.

Naidoo, J. & Wills, J. (2000) *Health Promotion – Foundations for Practice*, 2nd edn. London: Bailliere Tindall and Royal College of Nursing.

Shipman Enquiry: Fifth Report (2004) *Safeguarding patients: lessons from the past – proposals for the future*. Command Paper Cm 6394.

Tarrier, N., Haddock, H. & Barrowclough, C. (1998) Training and dissemination: research to practice in innovative psychological treatments for schizophrenia. In: T. Wyes, N. Tarrier & S. Lewis (eds), *Outcomes and Innovation in Psychological Treatment of Schizophrenia*. New York: John Wiley & Sons.

Index